# Legal and Ethical Aspects of Anaesthesia, Critical Care and Perioperative Medicine

**Dr Stuart M. White** FRCA BSc MA
Consultant in Anaesthesia, Brighton and Sussex
University Hospital Trust

**Dr Timothy J. Baldwin** BSc ARCS PhD LLB MA
Barrister of Lincoln's Inn
Visiting Lecturer in Law, School of Law, King's College London
2 Garden Court, Middle Temple, London

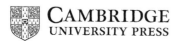

CAMBRIDGE
UNIVERSITY PRESS

PUBLISHED BY THE PRESS SYNDICATE OF THE UNIVERSITY OF CAMBRIDGE
The Pitt Building, Trumpington Street, Cambridge, United Kingdom

CAMBRIDGE UNIVERSITY PRESS
The Edinburgh Building, Cambridge CB2 2RU, UK
40 West 20th Street, New York, NY 10011-4211, USA
477 Williamstown Road, Port Melbourne, VIC 3207, Australia
Ruiz de Alarcón 13, 28014 Madrid, Spain
Dock House, The Waterfront, Cape Town 8001, South Africa

http://www.cambridge.org

First published 2004

Printed in the United Kingdom at the University Press, Cambridge

Typeface: New Baskerville 10.5/13pt    System: QuarkXpress®

*A catalog record for this book is available from the British Library*

ISBN 1 841 10209 1

The publisher has used its best endeavors to ensure that the URLs for
external websites referred to in this book are correct and active at the
time of going to press. However, the publisher has no responsibility for
the websites and can make no guarantee that a site will remain live or
that the content is or will remain appropriate.

Every effort has been made in preparing this book to provide
accurate and up-to-date information that is in accord with accepted
standards and practice at the time of publication. Nevertheless, the
authors, editors and publisher can make no warranties that the
information contained herein is totally free from error, not least
because clinical standards are constantly changing through research
and regulation. The authors, editors and publisher therefore
disclaim all liability for direct or consequential damages resulting
from the use of material contained in this book. Readers are strongly
advised to pay careful attention to information provided by the
manufacturer of any drugs or equipment that they plan to use.

# Legal and Ethical Aspects of Anaesthesia, Critical Care and Perioperative Medicine

on or before

Perioperative medicine and critical care are among the most litigious areas of medicine. The recent failure of doctors to convincingly resolve ethical issues concerning the morality of increasingly technological treatment has led to a diminution of trust in the medical profession by both the public and politicians, and a correspondingly rapid evolution of medical law.

This book, aimed at doctors, medical students, allied health professionals and lawyers, provides straightforward but detailed analyses of the ethical issues raised by many aspects of perioperative care and intensive medicine, and describes with clarity the current UK law governing such dilemmas.

Dr. Stuart White is a Consultant in Anaesthesia at the Royal Sussex County Hospital, and received an MA in Medical Law and Ethics from King's College, London. He is also an Honorary Lecturer in Medical Law at the University of Wales College of Medicine.

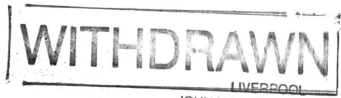

For
Cheryl, Ruari and Finn

# Contents

# 1

# Introduction

Medicine evolves. The human life cycle – birth, reproduction, death – is unremitting, but technological and social advances mean that not only do personal and societal patterns of disease change continuously, but also does our ability to cure or ameliorate disease. Indeed, the definition of 'disease' still remains a controversial concept.

The most notable feature of medical progress over the last 30 years is that its rate of evolution has markedly increased. There may be any number of reasons for this, including (but not limited to) improvements in information technology, the demand-led ethos of Western consumerism, the medicalisation of certain human conditions and behaviours, refinements and developments in scientific methods, and various political agendas relating to healthcare.

For decades, centuries even, the moral principles of Western medicine were informed primarily by the teachings of the classical philosopher-scientists, namely Thales, Hippocrates and Galen. These ideas were modified by the prevailing philosophical doctrines of subsequent historical periods: mainly religion before the Renaissance, humanism in the Age of Reason, and theories of Human Rights that have developed since the Age of Enlightenment. However, in our post-modern, secular society, there is growing concern that the recent accelerated rate of medical advance has outstripped the rate at which consequent ethical dilemmas can be discussed, or resolved. In particular, rapid advances in certain fields (e.g. in genetic engineering) mean that new moral dilemmas arise where there has previously been minimal, or no, ethical debate.

The simple question that arises is: why not just let medical progress advance unchecked by ethical scrutiny? Surely the ultimate goal of medicine is the alleviation of all disease and illness, and therefore medical progress is justification in itself? Indeed, many people might agree with this observation, and it may be difficult to see any other point of view when, for example, one is dying of a disease for which researchers are close to finding a cure. The simple answer is that there must be a right and moral thing to do. But can such a position really be maintained when one allies the subjective notion of 'doing the right thing' to research methods such as those used, for example, by some doctors under the Nazi regime? Or if one's chance of a cure necessarily entailed the death or disablement of another person? These dilemmas are the fundamental questions in medical ethics, namely that there are certain moral boundaries that cannot and (arguably) should not be crossed by individuals or society, that just because a treatment can be administered does not mean that it should be, and that the practice of medicine is so very much more than the application of a rationally scientific solution to a pathophysiological problem.

The failure of the medical profession to convincingly resolve ethical issues that have arisen has resulted in a diminution of trust in the medical profession by both the public and politicians, and a correspondingly rapid evolution of medical law, in order to circumscribe what society is currently willing to accept as 'ethical medical practice'. Of course, other factors have been influential in the development of medical law: medical consumerism emphasises patients' rights (further reinforced by statutory provision in the form of the Human Rights Act, 1998), the burgeoning body of case law progressively delineates acceptable medical practice in a self-propagating fashion, and politically-motivated anti-professionalism seeks to regulate medicine as a profession. Furthermore, there is a general expectation (through improved education via the media) that patients will not only receive healthcare as part of the welfare state, but that the standard of that care will be of an acceptable or highest attainable level; medical law regulates the reality gap between such demand and its supply. In addition to these factors, the acute, interdisciplinary nature of critical care and perioperative medicine, with their reliance on multiple, high technology interventions mean that these areas of clinical expertise are amongst the most litigation-prone in medical practice. The increased threat of litigation has, it appears, led to a concurrent rise in defensive medical practice; this has been beneficial in improving quality assurance in medicine, but has inevitably led to increased financial costs, distorted clinical decision-making and over-treatment of patients.

Uncertainty is an inherent component of evolution. Medical law and ethics are not immune to this. For example, we just don't know what the consequences of cloning humans, human stem cells or animals are going to be; we cannot foresee how the possible legalisation of physician-assisted suicide might alter society's attitudes towards the medical profession. However, by applying ethical principles to the moral predicaments, we might at least be able to decide what is and is not acceptable. Even then, this may not be the case: issues surrounding the practice of abortion, for example, are notorious for polarising peoples' attitudes. The effect of medical law is to resolve these issues one way or another (whether 'rightly' or 'wrongly'), so that at least decisions are made and boundaries set, and clinicians are informed in their day-to-day practice.

Medical law and ethics are currently 'hot topics' in the field of medical education. As discussed above, the plethora of ethical issues that have arisen from rapid scientific progress require extensive investigation and discussion. Whilst a considerable number of philosophers and allied professionals build their careers on so doing, there is an increased realisation that other interested parties, including doctors themselves, nurses and other health care providers, as well as patients and the general public would like to become – and should become – involved in the debate. Furthermore, the General Medical Council (GMC) has emphasised that all medical students should receive education in medical law and ethics as part of the core curriculum. In 1998, a consensus statement by teachers of medical ethics and law in UK medical schools reiterated the need for education in medical law and ethics in order to facilitate 'the creation of good doctors who will enhance and promote the health and medical welfare of the people they serve in ways which fairly and justly respect their dignity, autonomy and rights', and identified that these goals could be achieved through:

- ensuring that students understand the ethical principles and values which underpin the practice of good medicine;
- enabling students to think critically about ethical issues in medicine, to reflect upon their own beliefs about ethics, to understand and appreciate alternative and sometimes competing approaches and to be able to argue and counter-argue in order to contribute to informed discussion and debate;
- ensuring that students know the main professional obligations of doctors in the UK as endorsed by the institutions which regulate or influence medical practice particularly those specified by the GMC;
- giving students a knowledge and understanding of the legal process and the legal obligations of medical practitioners sufficient to enable them to practise medicine effectively and with minimal risk;
- enabling students not only to enjoy the intellectual satisfaction of debates within medical ethics and law but also to appreciate that ethical and legal reasoning and critical reflection are natural and integral components in their clinical decision-making and practice;
- enabling students to understand that ethical and legal issues arise not only in extra ordinary situations in medicine but also occur in everyday practice.

Aspects of the core curriculum include consent, confidentiality, research, abortion, death and the dying patient, rights, professional regulation and resource allocation, and these are the core chapters of this book.

Medical education traditionally dictates an allegiance to professional orthodoxy, such that 'doctors do this because that is how doctors do it, and have always done it'. The often abstract nature of medical ethics, with its emphasis on thought experiments and philosophical reasoning, can come as somewhat of a shock to the student. It is frustrating to the scientifically trained mind to conclude that there may not be a right answer (or even *any* answer!) to a problem. This book makes no apologies for not always stating what the current orthodoxy is. Instead, both by highlighting differing ethical viewpoints, and by providing the reader with the philosophical instruments on which to find an argument, it hopes to act as a springboard through which the reader might arrive at their own conclusions. The reader should not be surprised to note that there may be considerable dichotomy between their personal and professional ethics.

In terms of medical law, this book is more descriptive. Although there is considerable scope for the interpretation of legal decisions, it is usually of more value to those who are not legally trained to avoid conjecture and abstruse discussion, in favour of stating exactly what the law is. The dynamic nature of the subject, however, inevitably means that the law may have changed between the writing and publication of this book, and for this the authors apologise in advance. Recent decisions and reinterpretations of the law may be found in the *Medical Law Review* (http://www3.oup.co.uk/medlaw/).

## FURTHER READING

### Journals

Consensus Group of Teachers of Medical Ethics and Law in UK Medical Schools. Teaching medical ethics and law within medical education: a model for the UK core curriculum. *J Med Ethics* 1998; **24**: 188–192

Doyal L and Gillon R. Medical ethics and law as a core subject in medical education. *Br Med J* 1998; **316**: 1623–1624

### Book

General Medical Council. *Tomorrow's Doctors*. GMC, London, 1993

# 2

# An introduction to the UK legal system

Similarly to the other professions, the legal profession has established its own hierarchy, language and code of practice, in order to manage the large number of people professing general and specialist legal knowledge. As a result, the workings of the legal profession can appear arcane to the outsider, even despite recent attempts to improve public accessibility to the law.

This chapter provides a short introduction to legal system in the UK, as well as listing a number of sources of information by which the lay person may further access legal information.

## STRUCTURE OF THE UK LEGAL SYSTEM

The UK has three distinct legal jurisdictions: England and Wales, Scotland, and Northern Ireland. All of the jurisdictions are common law jurisdictions, but Scotland has a very distinct, separate and interesting legal system that incorporates aspects of the civilian system of law seen in continental Europe.

The legal profession in the UK is split into two branches, solicitors and barristers, whose training, practice and regulation are separate.

Solicitors are the legal equivalent of general practitioners, and are visited first by clients seeking legal advice. Solicitors instruct barristers to provide specialist legal advice and representation (if necessary) in court. Solicitors in England and Wales are regulated by The Law Society of England and Wales. In other countries of the UK they are regulated by the equivalent body.

Barristers play a similar role to that of hospital consultants, acting as a referral service for solicitors. They are the only members of the legal profession allowed to appear in the Appeal Courts and (in most cases) in the High Court. Most specialise in particular areas of the law, for example, clinical negligence. Barristers are not allowed to have direct access to lay clients, except in very limited circumstances, hence the requirement for

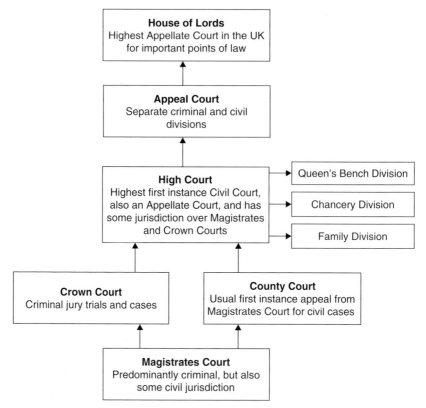

**Figure 2.1** The Court structure in the UK.

their instruction via solicitors. The activities of Barristers are regulated by the Bar Council of England and Wales. In the other countries of the UK they are regulated by the equivalent body.

The courts are administered by the Court Service under the Department of Constitutional and Administrative Affairs.

The fundamental distinction in the English common law is between Criminal Law and Civil (i.e. Non-criminal) Law. The court structure reflects this (Figure 2.1).

At the time of writing, as part of its Constitutional Reform Bill, the UK government is considering abolishing the role of the law lords in the House of Lords, in favour of a US-style Supreme Court. The Supreme Court would act as a final Appellate Court in the UK. Although this move is designed to reinforce the independence of the judiciary from political interference, critics have suggested that the current system has worked well for centuries and is delivered at a tenth of the proposed cost of the new system.

The Privy Council, one of the oldest parts of the government, maintains a judicial authority through a committee known as the Judicial

Committee of the Privy Council. This body is composed of Privy Councillors (life-appointments), for those who hold, or have held, high judicial office in the UK. The Committee hears appeals from those Commonwealth countries who have retained the right of appeal, from colonial territories and, importantly, from tribunals of the medical, dental and optician's professions.

Judges and tribunal lawyer members are appointed by the Lord Chancellor, who heads what used to be known as the Lord Chancellor's department, which has transformed itself into the Department of Constitutional Affairs (http://www.dca.gov.uk/index.htm).

In the Civil Courts the introduction of a completely new set of Civil Procedure Rules (April 1999), covering the procedure of the High Court and the County Court, is supposed to simplify court proceedings by giving judges more control over proceedings, and encouraging parties to settle their differences, preferably before litigation even starts. The rules also encourage the use of plain English in legal documentation.

The law of England and Wales is based on judge-made common law (or 'case law') based on court decisions ('precedents') made over a number of centuries, but is increasingly overlaid by a number of statutes (Acts of Parliament) and statutory instruments (secondary legislation that also has to be approved by Parliament). However, statute requires court interpretation, the decisions of House of Lords, the Court of Appeal and the High Court each being binding on the courts at lower levels. Decisions of the County Court are not normally reported and are only 'persuasive', (i.e. are not binding on other County Courts).

A further distinction that is made is between public law (pertaining to government and society) and private law (pertaining to disputes between individuals, also called civil law). Both public law and private law depend on statute and common law. The majority of public law relates to criminal law, compared to private law, which mainly concerns civil offences.

## THE EUROPEAN COURT OF JUSTICE

Membership of the European Union (EU) has added another layer of jurisdiction to the legal process of the UK.

Set up in 1952, the European Court of Justice (ECJ) acts as a Supranational Court (based in Luxemburg) that is able to enforce European Community (EC) law against individual defaulting EU Member States.

The ECJ comprises 15 judges and 8 advocates general. The judges and advocates general are appointed by common accord of the governments of the Member States and hold office for a renewable term of 6 years.

One of their numbers is selected by the judges to be President of the Court for a renewable term of 3 years. The President directs the work of the Court and presides at hearings and deliberations.

Judges ensure that EC law is not interpreted and applied differently in each Member State. In order to fulfil that role, the ECJ has jurisdiction to hear disputes to which the Member States, the Community institutions, undertakings and individuals may be parties. If it is judged that a Member State has not fulfilled its obligations under the Treaty of Europe, the Commission can initiate proceedings that require the State concerned to submit a defence of its position. If this fails to satisfy the Commission, a reasoned opinion may be delivered which requires the matter to be resolved by a specific date.

More than 500 cases are heard a year. To cope with the turnover of cases efficiently, a Court of First Instance has been set up by the European Council, whose advocates general assist the ECJ in its task, by delivering impartial and independent opinions on cases brought before the Court.

With relevance to perioperative medicine the ECJ may be asked to rule, for example, on the free migration of doctors between member states, on the application of the European Working Time Directive, on the right of individuals to become 'health-tourists' in order to facilitate more rapid access to treatment, and on the regulation of medicines and medical devices.

## THE EUROPEAN COURT OF HUMAN RIGHTS

The UK is bound by many international treaties which oblige it to respect human rights, in particular the European Convention on Human Rights (ECHR), a formulation of the Universal Declaration of Human Rights. This treaty allows those who believe their human rights infringed to appeal for redress to a higher court than that offered by the legal system of the UK.

The ECHR was drawn up under the auspices of the Council of Europe, an organisation of West European countries, based in Strasbourg, which is quite separate from the EC.

The rights guaranteed by the ECHR have recently been incorporated into UK statutory law as the Human Rights Act 1998 (see Chapter 4). In theory, this means that there will be fewer cases going to the European Court of Human Rights (ECtHR), as the UK courts should ensure adherence to the ECHR, although complainants may still be able to appeal to the ECtHR if, for example, they believe the law has been incorrectly applied.

There are two ways in which alleged breaches of the ECHR by the UK can be brought to the attention of the ECtHR:

- A complaint may be made by one of the other countries bound by the ECHR. In practice, countries are reluctant to bring cases against each other, doing so only in the most extreme cases or where their own interests are affected.
- More commonly, an individual may complain that his/her rights have been infringed. Any person claiming that their ECHR rights have been infringed may appeal directly to the ECtHR.

## GENERAL COMMENTS ON THE EVOLUTION OF MEDICAL LAW

Medical law is a comparatively young subject. Nevertheless, the continuing advance of medical technology, which often has debatable ethical consequences, together with the ongoing social development towards an increasingly consumerist society, has led to a boon in medicolegal practice. To an extent this is reflected by the previous paucity of legal guidance in the area. However, it may also represent enthusiasm on the part of the legal profession to extend the provisions of existing common law into the field of medicine, driven as much by financial reward as a crusading and altruistic desire to protect patients from the excesses of the medical profession. Whatever, medical law is here to stay, and will become a significant consideration in the professional lives of future doctors.

As mentioned, much of medical law has been guided by the courts, and decided by judges. However, increasingly, statutory provisions have been put in place by Parliament (e.g. the Human Fertilisation and Embryology Act, 1990). Nevertheless, the ethical dilemmas posed by medical advances tend to be avoided by politicians keen not to alienate potential voters, so it is likely that the courts will continue to provide the main guidance in the developing body of law, albeit modified and guided themselves by non-statutory but official edicts and guidelines from such august bodies as the British Medical Association (BMA), General Medical Council (GMC), and Department of Health.

## COURT TRANSCRIPTS AND HOW TO UNDERSTAND THEM

Consider the reference to the following judgement:

*ReF (in utero)* [1988] 2 All ER 193 (CA)

In this example, the case reference may be broken down into:

- *ReF*, which means 'in the case of *F*', *F* representing the first initial of the subject of the trial. *Re* usually precedes cases where a decision needs to be made about an individual, rather than more adversarial cases in which a decision needs to be made between parties (e.g. *Paton v Trustees of BPAS*). In the latter, the first name is the plaintiff or appellant (in the Court of Appeal) or claimant (in plain English). The second name is the defendant. *R v X* indicates a crown prosecution (i.e. *Rex (Regina) v X*), *A-G v X* indicates the involvement of the Attorney-General.
- *(in utero)*. Obviously, there are lots of people whose name begins with F. Bracketed terms in '*Re*' cases are an attempt to narrow the field of reference.
- [1988]. The year in which the case was reported, which is usually the same as the year in which the case was heard in court.
- 2. 2nd volume, etc.
- All ER. This describes the law report in which the case was reported. All ER: All England Reports; BMLR: Butterworth's Medical Law Reports; Med LR: Medical Law Review; Fam: Family Division Law Reports; EHRR: European Human Rights Reports; QB: Queen's Bench.
- 193. The first page of the report.
- (CA): the court before which the case was heard. CC: County Court; HCJ: High Court of Justice; Fam Div: Family Division; QBD: Queen's Bench Division; CA: Court of Appeal; HL: House of Lords; ECtHR: European Court of Human Rights, SC: Supreme Court (US, Canada and Australia).

Judges names are suffixed by the letters J (Justice); LJ (Lord or Lady Justice); MR (Master of the Rolls); P (President of the Family Court); LCJ (Lord or Lady Chief Justice); VC (Vice-Chancellor) and LC (Lord Chancellor). Judges in the lower courts are usually referred to as HHJ (His/Her Honour Judge).

## SOURCES OF INFORMATION ABOUT MEDICAL LAW AND ETHICS

There are, of course, any number of books, journals and web sites containing information about medical law and ethics.

The following references are good starting points, being both readable and easily accessible.

## MEDICAL ETHICS

### Books

Campbell A, Charlesworth M, Gillett G and Jones G. *Medical Ethics*, 2nd edition. Oxford University Press, Oxford, 1997

Glover G. *Causing Death and Saving Lives*. Penguin, London, 1977

Hebert PC. *Doing Right – A Practical Guide to Ethics for Medical Trainees and Physicians*. Oxford University Press, Ontario, 1996

Hope T, Savulescu J and Hendrick J. *Medical Ethics and Law – The Core Curriculum*. Churchill Livingstone, Edinburgh, 2003

Kuhse H and Singer P (Eds). *Bioethics – An Anthology*. Blackwell publishers, Oxford, 1999

Ridley A. *Beginning Bioethics*. St. Martin's Press, New York, 1998

Scott WE, Vickers MD and Draper H. *Ethical Issues in Anaesthesia*. Butterworth Heinemann, Oxford, 1994

Singer P. *Practical Ethics*, 2nd edition. Cambridge University Press, Cambridge, 1993

Steinbock B and Norcross A (Eds). *Killing and Letting Die*, 2nd edition. Fordham University Press, New York, 1994

### Journals

*Bioethics*
*Bulletin of Medical Ethics* (*Bull Med Ethic*)
*Journal of Medical Ethics* (http://jme.bmjjournals.com/) (hereafter: *J Med Ethic*)
*Journal of Medicine and Philosophy* (*J Med Phil*)

### Web sites

Bioethicsweb (http://www.bioethicsweb.ac.uk/)
Karolinska Institute (http://www.mic.ki.se/Diseases/K01.316.html)

## MEDICAL LAW

### Books

Jones MA and Norris A. *Blackstone's Statutes on Medical Law*, 3rd edition. Oxford University Press, Oxford, 2003

Kennedy I and Grubb A. *Medical Law*, 3rd edition. Butterworths, London, 2000

Mason JK and Smith MRA (Eds). *Law and Medical Ethics*, 6th edition. Butterworths, London, 2002

Montgomery J. *Health Care Law*, 2nd edition. Oxford University Press, Oxford, 2002

Partington, M. *Introduction to the English Legal System*. Oxford University Press, Oxford, 2003

## Journals

*British Medical Journal* (http://bmj.bmjjournals.com/) (*Br Med J*)
*Journal of Law, Medicine and Ethics* (http://www.aslme.org/pub_jlme/index.php) (*J Law Med Ethic*)
*Medical Law Review* (http://www3.oup.co.uk/medlaw/) (*Med Law Rev*)
*Medicine and Law* (*Med Law*)
*Medicine, Science and Law* (*Med Sci Law*)

## Web sites and legal search engines

All England Direct (requires Athens password)
BAILII
Butterworths
JUSTIS (requires Athens password)
Lawtel
LexisNexis
Statutory instruments – Her Majesty's Stationery Office (HMSO) (http://www.hmso.gov.uk)
The Medical Defence Union (http://www.the-mdu.com)
Westlaw

## Regulatory bodies

British Medical Association (http://www.bma.org.uk)
Department of Health (http://www.doh.gov.uk)
General Medical Council (http://www.gmc.org.uk)
Royal Colleges

## Medical search engines

Ingenta (requires Athens password)
Medline
PubMed
ScienceDirect (requires Athens password)

# 3

# An introduction to medical ethics

Ethics is a branch of philosophy that is concerned with how the individual may best lead a good life. Simply put, medical ethics is the application of ethics to the practice of medicine – namely how the clinician, or group of clinicians, might provide medical care to the best of their ability and for the maximum benefit of their patients, or society.

What constitutes the 'good life' and the practices which enable 'goodness' on the part of the individual have been the subject of philosophical debate for several millennia. The basis of Western ethical thinking was founded in the Greek city states from the 5th century BC onwards. At the time, philosophy was a communal affair, and great philosophers were also great orators. Socrates (469–399 BC) declared that morality is not concerned with obeying the law, more that a degree of introspection is needed such that once we know who we are, we will know how to lead a good life. His pupil Plato (428–354 BC), in *The Republic*, extensively discusses the nature of justice and the nature of the ideal State, his work underpinning much of Western philosophy for the next 2000 years. In turn, Plato's pupil Aristotle (384–322 BC), in the *Nichomachean Ethics*, introduced a measure of pragmatism to moral thinking, declaring humans to be born with the potential for goodness, but requiring us to discover what it is to be good through the application of common-sense (which is arguably the method by which much of UK common law is still derived). Little changed for the next 1500 years; Christianity, rather than reject the teachings of the Greek philosophers, actively assimilated their writings into Christian morality (notably in the writings of St. Augustine (354–430) and St. Thomas Aquinas (1224–1274)). The eventual schism between church and state during the Renaissance and later the Reformation gave rise to a more humanist approach to ethics, rejecting the notion of 'natural' (God-given) law in favour of the view that morality is a notion decided by humans. Thomas Hobbes (1588–1679), in *Leviathan*, introduced the idea of the 'social contract', which (rather pessimistically) pointed out that morality developed in such a way that essentially unpleasant human beings avoided harming each other. Jean-Jacques Rousseau

(1712–1778), on the other hand, preferred to think that humans were born with enormous potential for goodness, but required education to maximise that potential. In time, humanism gave rise to the two great moral theories that inform the ethical practice of modern medicine: utilitarianism (Jeremy Bentham (1748–1832) and John Stuart Mill (1806–1873)), and deontology (Immanuel Kant (1724–1804)), which are discussed in greater detail below.

Throughout the period described above, Western medicine was also developing. Similarly to the practice of philosophy in the Greek city states, medicine was a communal affair, directed by philosopher scientists such as Thales (640–546) and Hippocrates (460–370 BC). It was the latter, of course, who is credited with first describing the application of morality to the practice of medicine, in the Hippocratic Oath (Figure 3.1). Interestingly, there is little evidence to support the idea that Hippocrates himself wrote the Oath, and there are several inconsistencies between the affirmations and prohibitions in the Oath and other writings attributed

---

I swear by Apollo the physician, and Aesculapius, and Hygeia, and Panacea and all the gods and goddesses, making them my witnesses, that I will fulfil, according to my ability and judgment, this Oath and covenant:

*To hold him, who has taught me this art, as equal to my parents, and to live my life in partnership with him, and if he is in need of money to give him a share of mine, and to regard his offspring as equal to my brothers in male lineage, and to teach them this art if they desire to learn it without fee and covenant; to give a share of precepts and oral instruction and all the other learning to my sons and to the sons of him who has instructed me, and to pupils who have signed the covenant and who have taken an oath according to the medical law, but to no one else.*

*I will apply dietetic measures for the benefit of the sick according to my ability and judgment; I will keep them from harm and injustice.*

*I will neither give a deadly drug to anybody if asked for it, nor will I make a suggestion to this effect. Similarly I will not give to a woman an abortive remedy. In purity and holiness, I will guard my life and my art.*

*I will not use the knife, not even on sufferers from stone, but will withdraw in favour of such men as are [skilled] in this work.*

*Whatever houses I may visit, I will come for the benefit of the sick, remaining free of all intentional injustice, of all mischief, and in particular of sexual relations with both male and female persons, be they free or slaves.*

*What I may see or hear in the course of treatment or even outside of the treatment in regard to the life of men, which on no account [ought to be] spread abroad, I will keep to myself, holding such things shameful to be spoken about.*

If I fulfil this Oath and do not violate it, may it be granted to me to enjoy life and art, being honoured with fame among all men for all time to come; if I transgress it and swear falsely, may the opposite of all this be my lot.

---

**Figure 3.1** The Hippocratic Oath.

to Hippocrates (notably, the prohibition of abortion by the Oath). Nevertheless, the Oath has retained its primacy as the code by which physicians practice medicine right up to the modern day, albeit in a number of re-edited formats according to the prevailing societal *mores*.

The Hippocratic Oath describes a number of affirmations (e.g. treating patients to the best of one's ability, providing education to students free of charge), and a number of prohibitions (e.g. not to kill or harm patients, not to take part in abortions, not to form sexual relationships with patients, not to divulge confidential information). However, whereas the Oath provides general guidance about how physicians should conduct themselves professionally, there is little in the Oath that remains applicable to the practice of modern medicine. Indeed, the Oath may comfortably be *précised* to the following:

'I swear that I will fulfil, according to my ability and judgment, this Oath and covenant:

> to give a share of oral instruction [to other doctors], to treat the sick according to my ability and judgment; I will keep them from harm and injustice.
>
> I will neither give a deadly drug to anybody if asked for it, nor will I make a suggestion to this effect.
>
> I will remain free of all intentional injustice, and in particular of sexual relations with both male and female persons.
>
> What I may see or hear in the course of treatment or even outside of the treatment in regard to the life of men, which on no account [ought to be] spread abroad, I will keep to myself

If I fulfil this Oath and do not violate it, may it be granted to me to enjoy life and art; if I transgress it and swear falsely, may the opposite of all this be my lot'.

## SOME GENERAL POINTS ABOUT MEDICAL ETHICS

### Thinking about medical ethics can be very difficult for the scientifically-trained mind

Ethics often deals with abstract concepts that are impossible to prove. Not only can it be difficult to think about such concepts in a logical manner, but the articulation and communication of thought can prove to be torturous. There is considerable emphasis placed on thought experiment, which can lead to accusations by frustrated individuals that medical ethics has no place in the real world. For example, Judith Jarvis Thomson uses the wholly implausible analogy of a famous violinist who is surgically attached to a non-consenting kidnappee for 9 months, in order to defend abortion as an ethically acceptable practice (see Chapter 8). However, that the scientist cannot *prove* an ethical argument through rigorous experimentation misses the point: ethics is more concerned with what *should* happen, rather than what *does* happen.

## Medical ethics is not the same as medical law

What an individual physician *should* do is not necessarily the same as what the individual physician is required to do by law. However, there is a long tradition in developed countries that legal parallels have generally followed the morals adopted by society. For example, recognition of the moral wrongness of slavery in the 19th century resulted in the Abolition of Slavery Act, 1833; similarly, the Representation of the People Act, 1918 and the Abortion Act, 1967 were legal responses to the moral acceptance of the equality of female rights, and abortion.

Nevertheless, that a society legally sanctions certain activities does not automatically mean that those activities are morally acceptable. Numerous examples exist or have existed previously: medical involvement in the death penalty or State-sanctioned torture, the use of mentally ill patients for medical research purposes, and, more contentiously, the involvement of doctors in euthanasia. In the case of medical ethics, this dichotomy is most apparent when medical practitioners have a dual role, such that they are the patient's doctor but are also acting as an agent of the State, for example, by working as military doctors, for the prison service, or for the immigration service.

## Old ideas remain valid

Similarly to scientific theories, ethical theories and principles evolve, and are refined in line with new knowledge and debate, and with the development of new technologies (e.g. gene therapy). However, medical progress tends to continuously re-evaluate what is known in light of what scientifically provable, leading to the rapid rejection of hypotheses or ideas if they prove wrong, or are academically unsustainable. In contrast, there is less of a tendency in ethical thinking to reject ideas founded in antiquity: the moral theories of Kant and Mill, for example, remain valid today, albeit modified by extensive argument and counterargument.

## Relativism

It is often argued in modern society that 'immoral' means nothing more than 'contrary to the morals of a certain time and place'. The Spartans, for example, practiced active euthanasia – an alien concept to most 21st century Westerners; a relativist might argue, however, that contemporary abhorrence of active euthanasia might be similarly viewed as abhorrent by 23rd century moralists, because it denies a dignified death to certain individuals.

Latter day notions of individual rights tend to support and proliferate the idea of moral relativism, particularly the idea that it is wrong for certain individuals to foist their own moral codes on others: there is a degree of moral repugnance, for example, that 19th century imperialism imposed European moral values upon Africa (and other less developed nations), forcing the 'noble savage' (Rousseau) to abandon traditional moral codes and practices, to his detriment.

The problem with relativism is that it tends to accept all values and ethical standpoints as having equal moral worth. Numerous critics have pointed out, however, that relativism denies that there are any absolute moral principles. Cultural practices such as cannibalism, infanticide, euthanasia and female circumcision would therefore be considered as morally acceptable, merely because they form part of the value system of that culture. This cannot be the case: there should be certain moral principles that transcend cultural, religious or national borders, such that it is universally accepted that, for example, torture is *always* wrong.

In practice, pragmatism may confuse the issue still further. It is not relativistic, for example, to assert that torture is wrong *except under very specific circumstances* (e.g. to extract information from an individual in order to prevent a major terrorist atrocity, if this is the only method of gaining such information). Nor is this codicil an indictment of ethics *per se*, such that there is no such thing as an absolute moral truth. The basic idea here is that there are certain moral principles towards which good individuals and good societies should strive, the observance of which would remove the necessity for their transgression – in 'good' societies, situations necessitating the use of torture would simply never arise.

## Beware of slippery slope arguments

Slippery slope arguments are used to illustrate the possible consequences of an ethical standpoint. For example, a slippery slope argument used to reject active euthanasia may run as follows:

'active euthanasia is wrong. If society were to accept active euthanasia, then before long, we wouldn't just be providing a means of dignifying death for a few individuals: the floodgates would open, the boundaries would be pushed back, and it would become acceptable to kill the demented, the elderly, the physically disabled, criminals and political dissidents. Initially, people would be able to control the manner of their deaths; eventually, this autonomy will become eroded and doctors would be allowed to kill patients at will or according to financial considerations.'

Slippery slope arguments are powerfully emotive, but are often seriously flawed on two accounts:

- they are conjectural – what *may* happen is not necessarily what will happen,
- they are usually pessimistic in outlook, illustrating the worst case consequences rather than highlighting any beneficial outcomes.

Using the above example, it is equally valid – though still conjectural – to argue that:

'active euthanasia is currently regarded as wrong. However, if society were to accept active euthanasia, a number of the terminally ill would be empowered to choose the manner and time of their death, and would retain a measure of dignity in so doing. Implementation of such decision-making would have further beneficial consequences: it would go a long way to removing the suspicion held by the public that doctors either let patients die through omitting treatment, or covertly kill them through the administration of potentially lethal doses of painkilling drugs, thus improving trust in the medical profession; it would permit the reallocation of scarce resources away from the provision of terminal care towards the medical treatment of other patients; and it would compel the government of the day to legislate in this area, to put in place legal safeguards to protect both doctors and patients.'

## Religion

For much of the history of the Western world, 'ethics' has been synonymous with 'religious ethics', in that the prevailing social mores have been guided and regulated by religious doctrine. This state of affairs began to change after the Renaissance and with the rise of humanism, but religious dogma has continued to act as a potent source of moral direction even up to the present day. This is of course completely non-sensical: it is stifling to any debate about abortion, for example, for a critic to say that it is wrong just because a church leader or religious doctrine says it is wrong. That is not to say that various religions or religious groups should not inform contemporary opinions about medical ethics, merely that some form of argument other than that based around religious teaching is required by such groups, on which to found their opinion.

## ETHICAL THEORIES AND ETHICAL PRINCIPLES

Simply put, ethical theories are general perspectives from which particular ethical issues can be debated. The ethical theories that are commonly applied to moral dilemmas in medicine include deontology, utilitarianism, value theory and rights theory. These theories place different emphases on various criteria for decision-making. Deontology, for instance, emphasises the importance of duty when making decisions, whereas utilitarianism emphasises the importance of a decision having a good outcome.

## Ethical principles

The usefulness of an ethical theory depends for the main part on its ability to achieve a common set of goals, known as ethical principles. In their influential book, *Principles of Biomedical Ethics* (1979), Beauchamp and Childress identified 'principlism' as the ethical decision-making process which negotiates between four basic 'privileged' fundamental principles, on the one hand, and the unique nature of specific moral situations on the other. The four basic principles identified are:

1 beneficence,
2 non-maleficence,
3 respect for autonomy,
4 justice.

## BENEFICENCE

In medicine, the principle of beneficence guides ethical theories and doctors to do 'good', or more particularly, to do good for patients – to strive to act always in the patient's best interests. This principle allies itself closely with utilitarianism, in that the promotion of doing good should usually result in a good outcome occurring. The mere fact of providing useful treatment for patients fulfils the principle of beneficence.

However, beneficence requires that someone other than the patient (which is usually the doctor) has to make a judgment about what is to be considered 'good treatment', and whether 'doing good' to a patient is actually the best thing to do. For example, evidence-based best practice may dictate that it is more beneficial for patients to undergo epidural anaesthesia in addition to general anaesthesia for the purposes of total hip replacement. Nevertheless, the patient may be petrified of receiving epidural anaesthesia, and refuse treatment.

The example above introduces an important point: ethical principles do not operate in isolation. Respect for the patient's autonomy, for example, is an important co-principle in this instance, such that respecting the patient's refusal of treatment may do more good than trying to force an unwanted treatment upon him.

When there is concord between what is desired by the beneficent doctor and the autonomous patient, dilemmas are unlikely to arise. However, when these principles conflict, discussion is required in order to determine which principle is more compelling in the circumstances. An obvious example is the refusal of blood by a competent Jehovah's Witnesses, when blood transfusion is indicated by the nature of the surgical procedure proposed. Current ethical thinking tends to promote the principle of respect for autonomy over that of beneficence.

## NON-MALEFICENCE

Non-maleficence ('least harm') is a similar concept to the principle of beneficence, but deals with situations in which none of the outcomes of a treatment are likely to benefit the patient. In this case, the doctor should strive to do the least harm to the fewest people. Once again, the decision-making is left to the doctor, rather than the patient, or others. For example, a doctor may choose conservative treatment options in the case of a demented patient diagnosed as having pancreatic cancer, rather than subjecting the patient to palliative surgery.

Some commentators have argued that the principle of non-maleficence is an irrelevance in modern medicine (as all treatments tend to have at least some benefit), and remains little more than a recognition of the physician's historical duty under the Hippocratic Oath to 'do no harm'. Others have pointed out that non-maleficence represents core value of deontological medical ethics, and may in fact be of more moral importance than beneficence, in that doctors have a duty not to harm *anyone* (at least intentionally), but only a limited duty to be beneficent to more limited numbers of people. For example, doctors may be considered to have a duty to all perioperative patients not to withhold pain relief after bowel surgery, but have a more limited duty to actively provide thoracic epidural anaesthesia to subgroups of these patients.

## RESPECT FOR AUTONOMY

Autonomy confers the idea that individuals who are capable of exercising deliberate and meaningful choices that are consistent with their own values should remain in control of their decisions, because they are the only people who completely understand the implications of their decisions for their chosen lifestyle. Individual experience is unique, therefore only individuals could have experienced those life events, and developed those opinions, which form the basis of a truly autonomous decision.

Respect for autonomy requires doctors and other third parties (e.g. relatives and lawyers) to respect patients' decisions about their medical treatment, even if those decisions are at odds with medical orthodoxy or advice, or are likely to cause the patient harm. Respect for autonomy also imposes a duty on doctors to give patients adequate information on which to form their decisions.

Respect for autonomy is closely tied with civico-political notions of human rights (Chapter 4), such that the right to self-determination has a measure of legal protection under human rights legislation (at least in the Western world).

However, doctors' duty to respect autonomy raises several problems:

1  What should be done about patients who do not possess autonomy? The ethical (and legal) position involves the principle of beneficence, in that doctors should always strive to act in the patient's 'best interests' in these circumstances, but the question arises as to whom determines the best interests of an incompetent patient.
2  What happens if the patient makes 'bad' choices? For example, should respect for autonomy be maintained by doctors treating a septicaemic patient refusing antibiotic treatment? Furthermore, what role does illness play in the making of bad choices (or no choices at all) by patients?
3  What happens if the patient delegates their choice to others, for example, to doctors ('you decide, doc') or to relatives ('my wife thinks I should …')?
4  What happens if the patient asks for something illegal, or that is not in the doctor's ability to provide? Assistance with suicide or euthanasia is an obvious example.
5  What happens if respecting the patient's autonomy may bring harm to others? What should the doctor do, for instance, if a patient refuses to tell his wife (who is also the doctor's patient) that he has contracted HIV?

Paternalists see these dilemmas as insoluble consequences of unqualified respect for autonomy, that necessitate the involvement of knowledgeable third parties (usually doctors) to make beneficent proxy decisions for the patient. Paternalism prioritises a patient's best interests over their wishes.

However, libertarians ('pro-autonomists') are of the opinion that paternalism represents a deliberate attempt by a knowledgeable elite to limit personal rights and curb personal choice. Libertarianism prioritises the patient's wishes over their best interests, and counters the above objections by suggesting, amongst other things, that:

1 The temporarily incompetent may have previously indicated their autonomous wishes through an advanced directive, or through discussion with relatives (who may be considered the more appropriate repositories of any proxy decision-making capacity).
2 Patients can never make bad choices, only misinformed ones – it is the role of the doctor to inform patients correctly in order to optimise their autonomy.
3 Delegation of autonomy may be considered either a failure of communication and information provision, as in the point above, or a form of autonomy in itself, if patients are happy to let doctors decide for them.
4 Respect for autonomy is a two-way process – the patient must also respect the doctor's autonomy, and therefore is not entitled to ask from the doctor anything which the doctor cannot provide.

A further discussion of autonomy, partial autonomy and paternalism may be found in Chapter 5 of this book.

## JUSTICE

The principle of beneficence suggests that doctors should provide patients with the best treatments, and to the best of their ability. The principle of respect for autonomy empowers patients to ask for the best of treatment. However, it is an undeniable fact that the cost and demand for medical treatments vastly outstrips the finances available for their supply.

The principle of justice, by contrast, demands that doctors treat patients fairly. Two components of justice may be identified:

• Similar patients with similar illnesses should receive similar treatments. By this criterion, 'postcode prescribing' (where different patients in the UK have differing levels of access to medical care, according to the financial plans of their local health authority) would obviously not be considered 'just'.

- The allocation of limited resources (including buildings, time, money and manpower) should be made only after carefully considering the effects of this process on all the various recipients of resources. Reallocation of resources towards a new high-dependency unit, for example, may result in less money being provided for certain types of surgery, or to pay agency nursing staff, leading to bed-closures.

A fuller discussion of the role of 'justice' in the allocation of health care resources may be found in Chapter 13.

## Ethical theories

Ethical theories serve as prescriptive philosophical bases for resolving moral dilemmas. No one ethical theory is more 'correct' than any other, and each theory presents a number of philosophical problems in addition to providing answers. Ethical theories merely provide a set of guidelines that may be applied when debating moral issues.

|  | Deontology | Utilitarianism | Virtue theory |
|---|---|---|---|
| **Founders** | Immanuel Kant | Jeremy Bentham, John Stuart Mill | Aristotle |
| **Central concept** | An action is right if, and only if, it is in accord with a moral imperative | An action is right if, and only if, it produces the happiest consequences | An action is right if, and only if, a virtuous agent would perform the action in the circumstances |
| **Advantages** | • Consistent<br>• Acknowledges supererogation<br>• Concerned for justice | • Consequences of actions matter<br>• Benevolent<br>• Rational | • Actor matters more than action<br>• Pluralistic<br>• Codified |
| **Disadvantages** | • Indifferent to consequences<br>• Choice of rules may be irrational<br>• Rules may conflict | • Indifferent to justice<br>• Calculation of 'happiness' is irrational<br>• Inconsistent (act utilitarianism)<br>• Rules may conflict (rule utilitarianism) | • Egocentric<br>• Limited value in resolving ethical dilemmas in medicine |

**Figure 3.2** A summary of the three main ethical theories.

Three ethical theories have traditionally informed medical ethics:

- deontology,
- utilitarianism,
- virtue ethics.

Rights theory is discussed further in Chapter 4. Communitarianism as an ethical theory is also discussed below.

Recognition of the rather esoteric nature of these theories has encouraged modern medical philosophers to propose more pragmatic ethical theories, the most notable being consensus theory.

## DEONTOLOGY

'Deontology' (*Greek: deon-* duty; *logos* science, literally 'science of duty') refers to duty-based ethical systems, which hold that people act in a morally correct way when they act according to their duties and moral obligations, regardless of the consequences of their actions. Conversely, the deontologist may perform an ethically unacceptable action if he or she violates his or her duties or obligations, even if this action has a good outcome. For example, a doctor might have a duty not to betray a confidence about one patient to another, even if, were he to do so, he might prevent harm to the second patient. Individuals may act creditably above and beyond the call of duty ('supererogation'), but are not obliged to do so; for example, doctors may have a duty to provide intensive care treatment to certain patients, but are not obliged to provide the care without rest or holidays.

Nevertheless, simply following the correct moral rules is insufficient – in addition, individuals have to have the correct motivations, in order to allow a person not to be considered immoral even though they have broken a moral rule. 'Do not kill' may therefore be translated as 'do not kill, except in self-defence, or in order to defend those unable to do so themselves'. However, it is important to understand that correct motivation alone is not a justification for an action, and may not be used as to describe an action as morally correct. It is also insufficient to merely believe that an action follows a correct duty. Duties and obligations must be objectively determined, and are absolute in their nature.

Many traditional systems of ethics are deontological in nature, and usually prescribe a number of prohibitions. For example, Christian morality was founded around the Ten Commandments ('Thou shalt not kill', etc.), and medical morality was traditionally based on the Hippocratic Oath (see above).

The theory of deontology itself was formalized by Immanuel Kant (1724–1804). In *Fundamental principles of the metaphysics of morals* (1785),

Kant identified two types of obligation ('imperative'), which might inform people what to do in a moral dilemma:

- *Hypothetical* imperatives are conditional, such that actions should be performed in order that a goal might be achieved: medical treatment should be provided in order to make the patient better.
- *Categorical* imperatives are unconditional rules, and act as universal truths: medical treatment should be provided, because medical treatment should be provided.

Kant suggested that categorical imperatives were of the utmost importance: the only system of morals worth subscribing to depended on a rational society deciding (through pure reason) which rules should apply universally to the actions of all people. Kant proposed a number of categorical imperatives, the most famous of which is 'people should not be treated as a means to an end'. For example, doctors should not deliberately harm research patients in order to find out the side-effects of a drug, even if this will prevent similar harm occurring to patients in future.

Several types of deontological systems have been described:

- *Contractualism*: an action is morally right if it accords with the rules that rational moral agents would agree to, if they were entering into a 'social contract.'
- *Divine command*: an action is morally correct if it accords with rules handed down by God.
- *Duty theories*: an action is morally right if it accords with a specified list of duties and obligations (Hippocratic Oath, Kantianism).
- *Monistic deontology*: an action is morally right if it accords with some single deontological principle which guides all other subsidiary principles.
- *Rights theories*: an action is morally right if it respects universal human rights.

Although deontology contains many positive attributes, a number of theoretical weaknesses have been noted:

- Individual duty is seldom determined in a logical fashion. A surgeon may decide, for example, that it is always his duty to arrive in theatre 10 min before the start of an operating list, even if he is unable to rationalise exactly why this should be the case.
- An individual's duties may conflict. What is the surgeon to do, for example, if his duty to provide emergency resuscitative treatment to a patient on the ward prevents him from fulfilling his duty to arrive in theatre 10 min before the start of his operating list? Furthermore,

what are the criteria that he should use to resolve this conflict of duty? (Under such circumstances, it has been suggested that the individual should go on to consider the consequences of conflicting duties, and then judge which is the most '*prima facie*' of these.

• Deontology appears to be indifferent to the consequences of performing specified actions, which may harm others. For example, if the surgeon decided that he had a more pressing duty to arrive in theatres 10 min before the start of his operating list, the ward patient could suffer as a consequence. However, some critics have argued that, in practice, deontology has evolved into a form of consequentialism, in that commonly accepted duties are actually those actions which have been demonstrated over long periods of time to have the best consequences.

## UTILITARIANISM

Utilitarianism is one of a number of consequentialist ethical theories. Consequentialsim stresses that it is the consequences of an individual's actions that matter in the moral sense. In the case of utilitarianism, an action has moral value if it produces the most happiness, and is morally wrong if it produces the opposite of happiness.

Utilitarianism relies on both the ability to foresee the consequences of an action, and to allocate quantifiable units of intrinsic value to an action or consequence. Utilitarian consequences summate all of the happiness and unhappiness produced during the action, or arising as a consequence of the action. As a result the utilitarian can compare similar predicted solutions, and can determine which choice is the most beneficial to the most people.

Normally, a best course of action will make itself clear, although actions are only described as 'right' or 'wrong' if the consequences are of such significance that an individual feels compelled, rather than merely persuaded, to perform that action. If no clear benefit through either action becomes apparent, however, the utilitarian is not compelled to decide between them, according to his or her sense of morality, but merely according to which action is calculated to have the best consequences. For example, on the basis of mortality statistics, a utilitarian doctor might stop providing intensive therapy for octogenarians in order to reallocate resources to young polytrauma victims. However, the happiness afforded the younger patients (through possibly improved survival and rehabilitation) might be calculated to narrowly outweigh the unhappiness attributable to the older patients (mortality further increased, sense of injustice and contravention of human rights), which would render the wider moral issues raised by such resource reallocation irrelevant to the utilitarian.

Utilitarianism was formally developed by Jeremy Bentham (*Introduction to the Principles of Morals and Legislation* (1789)) and John Stuart Mill (*Utilitarianism* (1861)). Mill wrote of utilitarianism:

'The creed which accepts as the foundation of morals, utility or the greatest happiness principle, holds that actions are right in proportion as they tend to promote happiness, wrong as they tend to produce the reverse of happiness. By happiness is intended pleasure and the absence of pain; by unhappiness, pain and the privation of pleasure'.

Two types of utilitarianism are recognized:

- Act utilitarianism adheres precisely to the definition of utilitarianism, in that individuals are compelled to perform actions that benefit the most people, without regard to personal rights or feelings, or the societal restrictions, such as the law. Act utilitarianism has been described as hedonistic utilitarianism.
- Rule utilitarianism is less absolute, acknowledging that the best consequences are often contingent on notions of justice and social constraint. Rule utilitarianism seeks to maximise welfare, but only through fair and just means.

Although utilitarianism contains many positive attributes, a number of theoretical weaknesses have been noted.

- Happiness is more than an objective quantity. Furthermore, different people in different circumstances may experience differing amounts of pleasure. A patient diagnosed with a terminal illness, for example, may initially be terrified and depressed about their condition, before achieving a measure of acceptance and happiness with their remaining life, contrary to the degree of unhappiness that might be attributed to their condition by others. If happiness is not quantifiable, it is not possible to calculate the value of a consequence of action, and utilitarianism fails.
- The best consequences are not necessarily obtained by the most moral methods – 'the end does not justify the means'. It is not acceptable, for example, for doctors to transplant the hearts of patients in persistent vegetative state (PVS) into patients requiring heart transplant, even if the donor is considered as having no interests, the recipient survives and the surgeon benefits financially from the procedure.
- Utilitarianism may lead to injustice. If a first course of action produces 100 points of happiness for one person but 10 points of

unhappiness for eight other people, and a second course of action produces 10 points of unhappiness for the first person and 5 points of happiness for the other eight people, then the first course of action is the most utilitarian. However, this denies happiness to the majority, at the expense of an ecstatic minority. Conversely, for example, in deciding to spend money on either a screening programme for prostate cancer or a renal transplant service, a utilitarian may determine that the greatest good is being provided for the greatest number of people in the former instance, to the detriment of patients requiring renal transplantation. This is sometimes termed 'the distribution problem'.

- Utilitarian calculations do not place value on supererogation on the part of the actor. In other words, people are required to behave consistently, regardless of the circumstances. The utilitarian who sacrifices his life to save his friends is only seen as fulfilling a societal obligation, rather than acting in a selfless and laudable manner.
- Additionally, act utilitarianism is often inconsistent. When there is a change in the variables on which a decision is based, the act utilitarian may be forced to change their original decision.
- Rule utilitarianism also faces an additional problem, that there is the possibility of conflicting rules. The rule utilitarian anaesthetist who believes both that all patients should receive postoperative analgesia, and that all patients should have their autonomy respected, may face a dilemma if a patient refuses any form of postoperative pain relief after laparotomy.

## VIRTUE THEORY

Virtue theory focuses on the character of the individual, and judges any unusual and unethical action of that individual according to their morals, reputation and motivation. For instance, if a doctor refused to review a critically ill patient when invited to by a colleague, the colleague will be able to judge the action according to what he knows about the doctor's normal character. If the doctor normally follows the rules and is well respected amongst his colleagues, the colleague may be able to judge the doctor with greater lenience. Perhaps for example, the doctor has been otherwise busy, or there has been a breakdown of communication along the line. Conversely, a doctor who is well known for his laziness or indifference would be more likely to be judged unsympathetically by his colleague, because the doctor consistently lacks virtue.

Virtue ethics was developed by Aristotle, who indicated that a virtuous person (i.e. one who possesses the virtues) would always perform the right act according to the circumstances. The best life was to be had by possessing the virtues, leading to a state of *eudaemonia*, akin to the spiritual states described as 'heaven' or 'nirvana'. This is not so egocentric as it sounds: for example, doing good to and for others may be a by-product of a person's search for *eudaemonia*. Virtues commonly ascribed to the virtuous include courage, honesty, probity, humour, gravity, dignity, professionalism, humanity and equity.

Two weaknesses of virtue theory limit its application to medical ethics: firstly, the concept of virtue is rather nebulous and it remains uncertain whether the pursuit of virtue enables decision-making in any way. Secondly, virtue theory does not take into consideration a person's change in moral character. For example, the unhelpful doctor described previously may be undergoing a personality change at the time of referral, either from helpful to unhelpful or *vice versa*.

## COMMUNITARIANISM

Communitarianism rejects the individual and rights-centred approaches of the aforementioned ethical theories, and places the commonly agreed function of the community at the fore. Modern-day communitarianism began as a critical reaction to John Rawls landmark 1971 book *A Theory of Justice*. With reference to Aristotle and Hegel, political philosophers disputed Rawls' assumption that resources and liberties need to be distributed fairly in order to achieve free lives. No communitarian theory as such has ever been proposed, but these philosophers suggested, *inter alia*, that other factors should also carry weight when considering moral dilemmas, namely the importance of tradition and social context, the role the individual plays in society, the role society plays on the individual, the societal responsibilities of individuals and the value attached to belonging to a community.

Concerning medical ethics, it has been suggested that communitarianism underlies, or should encourage, for example, the practices of volunteering for research, presumed consent for organ donation, acceptance of waiting lists and rationing, and blood donation.

## CONSENSUS THEORY

The ethical theories and principles described above usually inform the decision-making process, each bringing their own attributes (and flaws) to the deliberation of moral dilemmas. However, critics have argued that often the ensuing discussion is long-winded, and fails to provide a coherent solution to a problem. As a result there has been recent interest in the search for a more immediately applicable framework for resolving moral dilemmas.

Consensus theories are a form of ethical pluralism, in that they seek to include and incorporate aspects of all other theories (including those mentioned above, plus medicalism, feminist theory, narrative theory and casuistry), which may all be viewed to some extent as interrelated anyway, in order to arrive at a harmonious solution to moral problems.

Three models may be identified:

- Clinical pragmatism seeks to guide health professionals in cases that pose specific moral problems in the practice of medicine.
- Ethics facilitation uses trained facilitators to guide discussions about ethical issues.
- Mediation aims to resolve conflicts or dilemmas through the involvement of a neutral third party, in order to help the parties in a dispute to reach a mutually acceptable agreement.

## ETHICAL ARGUMENT

The ethical theories described above provide standpoints from which the individual might argue his point, the principles aims around which to weave the theories. Nevertheless, a third element is required in order to thoroughly and rigorously scrutinise an ethical predicament, namely the physical process by which the problem is discussed. Four components of rational debate are commonly identified:

- *Questions of fact*: In the initial stages, debate can be rather emotional in nature. It is worth establishing the facts of the matter, and their definition, before any opinion is advanced. Later in any debate, it is worth re-establishing the facts, in case of their distortion during the course of discussion.
- *Fair-mindedness*: It is important both to respect and be sympathetic to other people's opinions, and to allow them to give voice to their opinions.
- *Rationality*: Valid reasoning requires that an argument is logically correct. Analysis of the problem should take into account the precise nature of the problem, and try to identify areas of agreement and of disagreement between individuals holding

opposing views. The ethical principles and theories advanced as the viewpoints accepted by interested parties should remain consistent.

- *Reflective equilibrium*: This essentially requires that individuals constantly re-evaluate their own position, according to logical analysis of their argument and incorporation of the viewpoints of others, until either an impasse, or more hopefully, an agreement is reached.

Chapter 2 of this book examined the structure of the legal profession, statute and the role of precedent in case law. This chapter has outlined the tools by which medical dilemmas may be analysed from a moral perspective. The remainder of the book seeks to examine how all of these general principles apply to more specific instances in the practice of perioperative medicine.

## FURTHER READING

### Books

Beauchamp T and Childress J. *Principles of Biomedical Ethics*, Oxford University Press, New York, 1979

British Medical Association. Medical ethics today: its practice and philosophy. *Br Med J* Publishing, London, 1993

Kuhse H and Singer P (Eds). *A Companion to Bioethics*, Blackwell publishers, Oxford, 1998

Ridley A. *Beginning Bioethics*, St. Martin's Press, New York, 1998. Part 1, pp. 1–69

Rachaels J. *The Elements of Moral Philosophy*, 3rd edition. McGraw Hill, Singapore, 1999

### Journals

Aulisio MP *et al*. Health care ethics consultation: nature, goals, and competencies. A position paper from the Society for Health and Human Values–Society for Bioethics Consultation Task Force on Standards for Bioethics Consultation. *Ann Intern Med* 2000; **133**: 59–69

Callahan D. Principlism and communitarianism. *J Med Ethic* 2003; **29**: 287–291

Clouser KD and Gert B. A critique of principlism. *J Med Philos* 1990; **15**: 219–236

Cookson R and Dolan P. Principles of justice in health care rationing. *J Med Ethic* 2000; **26**: 323–329

Davis RB. The principlism debate: a critical overview. *J Med Philos* 1995; **17**: 511–539

Gillon R. Do doctors owe a special duty of beneficence to their patients? *J Med Ethic* 1986; **12**: 171–173

Gillon R. Autonomy, respect for autonomy and weakness of will. *J Med Ethic* 1993; **19**: 195–196

McCarthy J. Principlism or narrative ethics: must we choose between them? *Med Humanit* 2003; **29**: 65–71

O'Neill O. Paternalism and partial autonomy. *J Med Ethic* 1984; **10**: 173–178

Pellegrino ED. The metamorphosis of medical ethics. A 30-year retrospective. *J Am Med Assoc* 1993; **269**: 1158–1162

Savulescu J. Rational non-interventional paternalism: why doctors ought to make judgments of what is best for their patients. *J Med Ethic* 1995; **21**: 327–331

Spriggs M. Autonomy in the face of a devastating diagnosis. *J Med Ethic* 1998; **24**: 123–126

Wiland E. Unconscious violinists and the use of analogies in moral argument. *J Med Ethic* 2000; **26**: 466–468

# 4

# Rights, and the Human Rights Act, 1998

The Human Rights Act, 1998 (HRA) came into force throughout UK on October 2nd, 2000. The HRA incorporated most of the Articles of the European Convention of Human Rights (ECHR) into domestic law. Until that time, both the state and the individual were notionally allowed to act with relative freedom in pursuit of their own interests, provided those actions were in accordance with statutory provisions and common law. The HRA introduced the principle that the action of the state and public bodies had to be justified in accordance with the limitations imposed by the ECHR. Moreover, the HRA introduced the concept of positive rights into UK legislation. The legal and moral position now is such that both the human rights of the UK citizen and the responsibilities of the UK state have become legally defined.

## ETHICS

Human rights are considered practicable, inalienable, moral claims attributable to any human being (by reason alone of being human) that ought to be respected and enforced by all, in order to ensure the political and civil freedoms of individuals. In theory a right is to be morally respected even if it goes against the common good (e.g. parental refusal of vaccination for a child) or is at odds with a specific duty (e.g. refusal of treatment when a doctor thinks treatment is in the patient's best interest). To interfere with the exercise of a right requires a clear demonstration that another right will be unjustifiably interfered with, when exercising the first right. Not all rights are considered absolute, with greater weight being given to certain rights rather than others: for example, the right to life is ranked as a higher order right than the right to vote in free elections.

Historically, the philosophy behind the concept of human rights can be traced back as far as 1780 BC, and the codes of Hammurabi. The existence and determination of a definition of human rights has eluded and divided, philosophers, politicians and scholars for many centuries. The Western understanding of individual human rights has been a gradual evolution of the theory of 'natural rights', derived and developed from the natural law doctrine of Aristotle (*Nichomachean ethics* (330 BC)) and the Greek Stoics. This states that human rights find their source in nature, such that certain rights are attributed to all human beings by the mere fact of being human.

In England, The Magna Carta (1215) delineated the relationship between the state and its citizens, but its legal tenets were only applicable to England, although its principles have been adopted by many other countries, for example the USA. John Lilburn and the Levellers produced a manifesto of personal rights in the 1640s, but its subsequent incorporation into a British constitution was rejected by Cromwell and Parliament. A Bill of Rights was passed in the English Parliament in 1689.

In the late 17th century, a 'natural rights' theory was promoted by the influential forefather of modern human rights, John Locke. Locke stressed that men (and women) have natural rights to 'life, liberty and property'. Society, Locke argued, resulted from a 'social contract' between humans who took on certain obligations in order to create a social situation in which they could best fulfil their natural rights. In the latter part of the 18th century, Thomas Jefferson rejected the idea of a natural right to property and formulated the rights-based American Constitution (1787) around the idea that 'all men are created equal, that they are endowed by their Creator with certain inalienable rights, that among these are life, liberty and the pursuit of happiness'. These sentiments were echoed 13 years later by the slogan of the French revolutionaries – 'Liberte, Egalite, Fraternite'.

However, that a person has a natural right to do anything means that, theoretically, (s)he does not have to respect the natural rights of others. Locke did not see this as a problem, as he considered human beings to be fundamentally social and rational beings. However, a contemporary of Locke, Thomas Hobbes, saw that humans with the strongest will were likely to become the dictators of what the rights afforded to the individuals of a society should be. Others, such as Jeremy Bentham and Karl Marx, entirely rejected the theory of natural rights. Bentham suggested that the 'real rights' attributable to individuals were a result of 'real law'.

In addition to 'natural' and 'real' rights theories, some philosophers have justified rights on the basis of religion, by pointing out that the major world religions advocate some aspects of human rights. Others have criticised this position, by stating that religious doctrine is no more than a list of duties, such that, for example, 'respect for life' is the product of 'do not kill'. It has been further been argued that 'Western' human rights, although acknowledging natural and religious rights theories, have evolved mainly as a result of the social changes brought about by the Enlightenment and Industrial Revolution. Current notions of human rights, therefore, are secular, rather than religious, in origin.

Primarily, human rights have been considered as political or civil claims, such that criticism of the human rights record of a country is usually linked to criticism of the incumbent political regime and of its repressive attitude towards rights to life, liberty, personal security and freedom of movement, together with its sanctioning of torture, cruel, inhumane or degrading treatment, arbitrary arrest and detention. Current political and civil rights are the descendants of natural rights, and are therefore known as 'first-generation' human rights. However, Marx and Engels argued that certain individual rights had to be suppressed in order that higher rights be afforded to mankind as a whole. In a socialist society, Marx argued that the primary development of cultural and socio-economic rights would create a classless society, culminating in political and civil rights. Ever since publication of *Kapital*, the basis of socio-economic right as human right has been consistently challenged, mainly due to the fact that such rights are only nation dependant and their enjoyment depends on the wealth of that nation – the individuals of poor countries would thus never achieve political and civil rights. Cultural and socio-economic rights, so called 'second-generation human rights' are therefore considered more as 'citizen's rights' rather than human rights. They include rights to the highest attainable standard of health, access to work, food, clothing, social security, housing, education and the benefits of scientific research. In Europe, we are well aware of the ECHR drafted by the Council of Europe to protect political and civil rights. However, what tends to be less appreciated is that the Council of Europe and the European Union (EU) also have draft charters of second-generation socio-economic rights. It is arguable that to the greater majority of the population of Europe and the rest of the world, second-order rights may, in practical terms, be of greater importance than the first-order rights.

The ideological distinction between first-generation rights, as adhered to by capitalist countries, and second-generation rights, adopted by socialist countries, was one of the more insoluble problems facing the creation of International Conventions on Human Rights, such that most post-war declarations recognise political, civil, socio-economic and cultural rights. The inclusion of Third World countries into global politics has led to the inclusion of other ideologies concerning human rights. This has led to the conception of a third-generation of rights – 'solidarity rights' – that urge solidarity with the less privileged in order to bring about both the fair redistribution of resources and the alleviation of suffering.

Therefore, it is generally accepted that human rights, in the conventional sense, are derivatives of natural rights and are granted simply by virtue of being human – 'To have a human right one need not be or do anything special, other than to be born a human being' (Donelly). However, this excludes any form of physical or mental action and some critics have argued that rights are entitlements that have to be claimed by an individual or group and be enforceable by law (Rosenbaum). Others disagree with this, suggesting that because other rights are legally enforceable (e.g. animal rights), human rights are not a form of legal right so much as a form of moral right. Cranston has elaborated this position, arguing that human rights differ from other moral rights by being 'the rights of all people, at all times and in all situations', which effectively excludes religious and cultural interpretations of rights. In addition, this idea rejects the concept that human rights are the fulfilled expression of human desires or preferences ('Ideally, no one should ever die as the result of war', therefore, 'war is a contravention of human rights'). Cranston has developed three criteria to apply to a right to test its qualification as a human right:

- *Practicability*: something cannot be a right if it cannot be claimed, which tends to exclude second-generation rights.
- *Universality*: that is the right can be enjoyed by everyone, everywhere, regardless of their sex, age, race, religion, financial and political situation. This includes the right to life and liberty, but also to food, shelter and health care.
- *Paramount importance*: by which the right to life and freedom from physical or psychological torture are precedent over other human rights.

The rapid expansion of modern human rights legislation resulted from international moral revulsion concerning the atrocities of the Nazis in World War II. The United Nations Declaration on Human Rights (UDHR), in December 1948, guaranteed various rights and freedoms for the individuals and institutions of a society. Legal weight was added to the UDHR in 1950, by the adoption of the ECHR, a treaty of the Council of Europe. The ECHR has a dual purpose: it provides the peoples of Europe with a set of defined civil and political rights, while maintaining a commitment to preserving democracy and the rule of law. Most of the rights enunciated in the Convention are viewed as qualified rights (as opposed to absolute rights) and may be infringed where there is a pressing social need, in the legitimate interests of democracy when authorised by law. The ECHR was drafted by British lawyers, and Britain was one of the first countries to sign the treaty, although it was one of the last signatories to incorporate the Convention into its national law. Initially, successive UK governments thought that both common law and statutory provisions of Acts of Parliament would protect the rights of British citizens. When this consistently failed to happen, the Convention became incorporated into domestic law under the HRA. Royal Assent was granted in 1998, but the HRA did not come fully into force until 2000, in order to allow public authorities the time to review their procedures and train their staff in relation to the provisions of the Act.

## LAW

### The relevance of the HRA to medicine

The HRA regulates the relationship between individuals and public authorities. Individuals who believe their human rights, according to the articles of the HRA, have been violated or that there is a threat of violation by a public authority, now have recourse to the UK courts to seek a legal remedy against the public authority. Prior to the incorporation of the Convention into domestic law, in order for an individual to enforce their human rights in law, they would have had to apply to the European Court of Human Rights (ECtHR) in Strasbourg, a lengthy and expensive process. This process was necessary because domestic law did not recognise a violation of human rights as a means to bring a claim against a public authority.

Public authorities, as defined by the HRA, include the Department of Health, health authorities, health trusts, primary care groups and the General Medical Council (GMC) (when acting as a disciplinary body). Organisations set up to protect the health care professions, for instance the British Medical Association and Royal Colleges, are not generally considered to be public authorities. However, cases such as *Poplar Housing v Donaghue* [2001] 3 WLR 183 and *R (on the application of Heather and others) v Leonard Cheshire Foundation and another* [2002] 2 All ER 936 demonstrate that the concept of a public authority can be quite fluid and remains poorly defined. Section 6(3) of the HRA defines a public authority as a public body discharging a public function. Thus it may be arguable in the future that bodies such as the Royal Colleges are public bodies if they discharge a public function, for example providing guidance on adopting certain paradigms *per* the *Bolam* test (Chapter 5).

Section 6 of the HRA states 'it is unlawful for a public authority to act in a way which is incompatible with a Convention right'. Breaches of obligations may give rise to challenges and compensation claims by plaintiffs. The duty of a public authority to an individual extends beyond the interaction with that individual. In certain circumstances, public authorities must take measures to ensure the protection of staff from human rights infringements that occur due to the actions of other people (e.g. physical and verbal abuse).

The HRA affects doctors and other healthcare professionals in two main ways. Public authorities, such as the National Health Service (NHS), employ doctors and health professionals and are therefore obliged to treat their employees in accordance with the HRA. However, as employees, doctors and other health professionals are representatives or agents of public authorities and are therefore obliged to respect the human rights of patients.

As they are currently formulated, codes of ethical medical practice are compatible with the HRA and the articles of the ECHR, such that good medical decision-making, in conjunction with respect for confidentiality and patient autonomy, is unlikely to contravene the new legislation. Treatment dilemmas will still arise, but, in future, their resolution will have to accord with the principles of the HRA. However, these principles are not set in stone. It may be legitimate to interfere with a right guaranteed by the ECHR under certain circumstances. The justification of this interference will usually be by reference to a contradictory article of the HRA, although the degree of interference should be proportional to the intended objective. For example, interference may be warranted if a life is immediately at stake, but not warranted in order to facilitate elective treatment. With some of the qualified rights, a right may be interfered with, if it is in accord with some overriding public interest. In addition, states are allowed a 'margin of appreciation', which confers them certain freedoms in evaluating public policy decisions in relation to human rights provisions and reflects the necessity of national courts enforcing their own democratic traditions. Therefore, decisions made in the courts of other European countries regarding human rights violations may not be directly applicable to UK law.

Initially, legal interpretation of the HRA is likely to be difficult, due to the infancy of the Act. Although there is a body of Strasbourg jurisprudence, a sufficient body of English case law has not yet been developed against which the human rights aspects of health care may be measured. Until case law develops, analysis of how the HRA might affect medical practice in the UK is often conjectural.

## The articles

The HRA incorporates 18 articles from the ECHR, but not all are relevant to the practice of medicine (e.g. Article 16 that restricts the political activities of aliens). Only Article 3 (Prohibition of Torture) and Article 4 (Freedom from Slavery) describe an absolute human right. Some rights are limited by explicit exceptions; for example, Article 5 (Right to Liberty and Security) states that 'Everyone has the right to liberty and security of person' but allows 'the lawful detention of persons for the prevention of spreading of infectious diseases, of persons of unsound mind, alcoholics or drug addicts or vagrants' (5(1)(e)). Other rights are more broadly qualified (e.g. Article 10 (Freedom of Expression), with justification of the fundamental right in 10(1) being provided for in 10(2)). The articles with most relevance to perioperative medical practice are Articles 2, 3, 5, 8, 9, 10 and 14.

---

**Article 2** (Right to Life)

1. *Everyone's right to life shall be protected by law. No one shall be deprived of his life intentionally save in the execution of a sentence of a court following his conviction of a crime for which this penalty is provided by law.*

---

Article 2 is divided into two parts. The first part, cited above, encompasses a positive obligation on the state and public authorities to protect the lives of its citizens in law. The second part provides that the state should not cause the death of any of its citizens except in very limited circumstances.

The 'right to life' has obvious relevance to end of life decisions. However, the article does not imply that one should always strive to prolong life. This point was clarified by Mr Justice Cazalet in the case of a 19-month-old child suffering from severe, irreversible cardiopulmonary disease, Dandy–Walker syndrome and lissencephaly. The parents of this child opposed the decision of a hospital paediatrician not to resuscitate the child in the event of cardiopulmonary arrest. Mr Justice Cazalet stated that 'there does not appear to be a decision of the European Court which indicates that the approach adopted by the English court in cases such as this is contrary to Article 2.' (*A NHS Trust v D & Ors* [2000] 2 FLR 677) The judge held in this case that non-resuscitation was in the best interests of the child.

Nevertheless, the right to life should be considered in decisions that involve the withdrawal of life-sustaining therapy. In the UK, patients have a right to medical treatment that prolongs their lives according to Mr Justice Laws, in *R v Cambridge Health Authority, ex parte* B [1995] 25 (BMLR) 5. However, the Court of Appeal in this case recognised that health authorities are entitled to make rational decisions concerning resource allocation. Thus, the ECHR allows states a margin of appreciation or discretion to determine the extent to which they are obliged to discharge their positive duties under Article 2. To avoid breaches of Article 2, withdrawing or withholding medical treatment must be in the best interests of the patient. Consideration of feeding and hydration as 'futile treatments' (that have no medical effect) may allow their discontinuation (*Airedale NHS Trust v Bland* [1993] AC 789). In an important decision, Dame Elizabeth Butler-Sloss, the President of the Family Division of the High Court, recently considered the effect of Article 2 in relation to the withdrawal of medical care and treatment from two patients with persistent vegetative state (PVS) (*NHS Trust A v M; NHS Trust B v H* [2001] 2 WLR 942). She held that 'Article 2 therefore imposes a positive obligation to give life-sustaining treatment in circumstances where, according to responsible medical opinion, such treatment is in the best interests of the patient but does not impose an absolute obligation to treat if such treatment would be futile'. This decision supports those made in similar cases prior to the implementation of the HRA (e.g. in *Bland, ReG* [1995] 2 FCR 46).

Advance directives ('living wills'), if fully informed, voluntarily given and made by a competent adult, may allow a person to forego their right to life, by refusing life-sustaining treatment (*per* Goff L, in *Bland*, see also *Re AK*). In future, it has been suggested that patients making advance directives should clearly state that they reject the right to life under Article 2. Those threatening, or having attempted, to take their own lives are usually assumed to be incompetent to make a valid end of life decision and should be resuscitated. That a person has a right to life does not, by extension, imply that they have a right to determine the nature of their death, however. The legality of assisted suicide under domestic law and by virtue of the ECHR, whether by a relative or physician, was clarified recently by the House of Lords and the European Court of Human Rights in the Diane Pretty ruling.

The withholding of life-saving treatment due to resource rationing may breach Article 2. Examples include inaccessibility of intensive care facilities, refusal of resuscitation on the grounds of age (also possibly in breach of Article 14) or chronic disease, prescription restrictions on the basis of cost and 'postcode prescribing'. In its defence of rationing, a public authority will have to show that policy decisions concerning resource allocation have considered Article 2 in a rational, transparent and non-discriminatory way. The courts themselves are reluctant to be drawn into arguments about health care rationing, preferring to leave such decisions to the remit of the government.

Doctors may not be in breach of Article 2 if, by their actions, they prevent harm to others. For example, a doctor may consider breaching patient confidentiality if (s)he believed that a patient who knew they were Human Immunodeficiency Virus (HIV) positive had deliberately failed to disclose this fact to a spouse.

---

**Article 3** (Prohibition of Torture)

*No one shall be subjected to torture or to inhuman or degrading treatment and punishment.*

---

Article 3 is an absolute right and allows no derogation. This right imposes a positive obligation on the state to minimise inhuman and degrading treatment within its borders and imposes an obligation not to inflict such treatment on its subjects. Various interpretations of Article 3 exist, however, depending on the definition of 'inhuman or degrading treatment'. Doctors have a duty to draw attention to cases of inhuman or degrading treatment. For example, one may be obliged to inform the appropriate authorities if one felt a patient had received grossly inadequate medical or nursing attention on a hospital ward or if the delay of an operation for logistical reasons had caused a patient undue pain or distress. Patient advocacy is particularly relevant for vulnerable groups, including children, the elderly, the mentally handicapped and the poor, who may be unaware that their rights have been violated or are unable to seek remedy for their complaints. Those undergoing experimental treatment are also vulnerable, and measures should be in place to discontinue treatment if it is found to be detrimental, on the basis that this would constitute inhumane treatment. Other instances of 'inhuman or degrading treatment' may include excessive preoperative fasting, failure to provide adequate analgesia, failure to provide substitution therapy for drug addicts both prior to and after surgery, failure to prevent awareness under anaesthesia, inappropriate early discharge from the intensive care unit or hospital ward and failure to respect the dignity of a patient throughout a theatre episode.

Administration of medical therapy to a competent adult without consent could, in extreme circumstances, be found to be in breach of Article 3

(*Herczegfalvy v Austria* [1992] 15 EHRR 437). Similarly, failure to respect an expressed wish or advance directive, such that a competent patient, who had expressed a refusal, received life-sustaining treatment may constitute a breach of Article 3 (*D v UK* [1997] 24 EHRR 423). However, Article 3 would not be breached if necessary therapeutic treatment was given in the best interests of an incompetent patient (e.g. hemiarthroplasty for an 80-year-old patient with Alzheimer's disease), unless it is known that if the patient had previously been competent namely comprehended, retained, believed and weighed information (*ReC, ReMB*), she would have expressly refused that treatment.

There is likely to be a greater onus on doctors to assess the *Gillick* competence (see Chapter 5) of children under 16, in order that issues of consent for operation may be resolved. Following the ruling in *Gillick* (*Gillick v West Norfolk and Wisbech Area Health Authority* [1986] AC 112 House of Lords (HL)), the courts recognised that children less than 16 years of age, who were found to be competent, could give their consent to a range of medical treatments, even if the treatment proposed was against their parents' wishes. This ruling should have two effects. First, under 16s who are *Gillick* competent are likely to have there autonomy respected to a greater extent, allowing them increased freedom to consent to operations. Secondly, the respect for the autonomous decisions of a *Gillick* competent child under 16 may be extended to cases in which the child is refusing treatment, particularly when it is felt that the treatment is inhuman or degrading. At present, refusals of treatment by *Gillick* competent minors (often involving the refusal of food by anorexics) are usually overruled by parents or the courts. Similarly, 16- and 17-year olds, who are rebuttably presumed to be competent, may refuse treatment (although the courts have been reluctant to endorse refusals of treatment that may result in death). However, appeal to the HRA might, for instance, allow a competent 15-year old to refuse a life-saving procedure because of the potential for future pain, suffering and interference with a 'normal' existence.

Article 3 may also apply to cases concerning rationing of health care, particularly if palliative or analgesic care is withheld. A judicial review of one NHS trust's decision to ration the administration of analgesics to a severely mentally handicapped woman was challenged by reference to Article 3.

A recent decision rejected a breach of Article 3 in relation to the discontinuation of medical treatment for those in a permanent vegetative state, holding that withdrawal of treatment is neither inhuman or degrading if the patient has no awareness that (s)he is being treated (*NHS Trust A v M; NHS Trust B v H* [2001] 2 WLR 942).

**Article 5** (Right to Liberty and Security)

1. *Everyone has the right to liberty and security of person. No one shall be deprived of his liberty save in the following cases and in accordance with a procedure prescribed by law:*

   *(e) the lawful detention of persons for the prevention of the spreading of infectious diseases, of persons of unsound mind, alcoholics or drug addicts or vagrants;*

Article 5 has greatest medical relevance to the detention of 'persons of unsound mind', the definition of which is yet to be rigidly delineated, but which precludes 'views or behaviours which deviate from the norm prevailing in society'. The HRA does not provide the authority to detain individuals, but states that one exception to the right to be free from detention occurs *when the law has decided* those of unsound mind should be detained. UK Mental Health Law falls broadly in line with the HRA, though sections of the Mental Health Act 1983 (MHA), are under review. Physicians called on to sedate violent patients in casualty departments ('chemical restraint') could find themselves in breach of Article 5, if the patient could prove that they were not of 'unsound mind' at the time of restraint. Similarly, the practice of using physical restraints, either to stop patients pulling out their tubes in intensive care or when applied to prisoners to prevent their perioperative escape, could contentiously be in breach of Article 5.

**Article 8** (Right to Respect for Private and Family Life)

1. *Everyone has the right to respect for his private and family life, his home and his correspondence.*
2. *There shall be no interference by a public authority with the exercise of this right except such as is in accordance with the law and is necessary in a democratic society in the interests of national security, public safety or the economic well-being of the country, for the prevention of disorder or crime, for the protection of health or morals, or for the protection of the rights and freedoms of others.*

This is perhaps one of the most welcome articles for the medical profession. Previously, English law provided no right to privacy but only a public interest in maintaining confidences. In the UK, patients have the legal right to access their own medical records (see Chapter 8), which requires public authorities (including doctors) to maintain high standards of note-keeping. In light of the HRA, disclosure of patient data to a third party is only possible with expressed consent of the patient (*MS v Sweden* [1997] 3 BHRC 248), unless there is a legal obligation to disclose or where it is decided 'necessary in a democratic society in the interests of national security, public safety or the economic well-being of the country, for the protection of health or morals, or for the protection of the rights and freedoms of others.' Such data includes NHS records and test results, including genetic and HIV tests. Similarly, there is a greater burden on doctors to take care when relaying verbal information about a patient.

Disclosure of information to a patient or parent may necessarily have to be increased in order to validate informed consent or to facilitate the resolution of difficult treatment decisions. The more American 'full disclosure' approach to informed consent would seem to provide improved defence against battery or negligence claims, compared to the English 'need to know/what the patient can understand' approach. However, the problem with the American approach is that it overburdens the decision-maker with unnecessary information and is very costly. The present status provides for a workable circumstance.

Parents or those with parental responsibility, have a clear right to be involved in medical decision-making when it concerns their childrens' life or health, on the basis that the decision affects their family life. By analogy, medical information may be discussed with relatives involved in decision-making about the treatment of their incompetent relative. This has obvious relevance to treatment decisions in intensive care. However, the decision by doctors to disclose information to relatives must be balanced against the individuals right to confidentiality and it must be remembered that, at present, no individual may exercise a power of consent on behalf of an adult who has become incompetent (this may change if the government's Draft Mental Incapacity Bill becomes law – see Chapter 5).

Article 8 has additional implications for both the conduct and reporting of medical research. Again, there is an issue concerning the degree of information disclosure for the validation of informed consent with regard to the participation of subjects in research. Intellectual property – hypotheses or the results of research – may be guarded by Article 8. The use of photographs of patients without their expressed consent or failure to protect the identity of a patient (e.g. in written case reports) may contravene Article 8. Physicians should question the practice of videoing resuscitation episodes or operative procedures, unless it is clear that consent has been obtained from the patient. Medical students and other observers should be encouraged to seek the consent of the patient before observing consultations or operations.

---

**Article 9** (Freedom of Thought, Conscience and Religion)

1. *Everyone has the right to freedom of thought, conscience and religion; this right includes freedom to change his religion or belief and freedom, either alone or in community with others and in public or private, to manifest his religion or belief, in worship, teaching, practice and observance.*
2. *Freedom to manifest one's religion or beliefs shall be subject only to such limitations as are prescribed by law and are necessary in a democratic society in the interests of public safety, for the protection of public order, health or morals or for the protection of the rights and freedoms of others.*

---

The freedom of belief as defined by Article 9 is an absolute right. However, other aspects of Article 9 are qualified. Health professionals may challenge the right of patients or parents to consent or refuse medical intervention, on the grounds of belief or religion, if intervention is in the best interests of the individual or necessary to preserve their life. In this respect, the HRA often supports existing English law. For example, doctors may challenge the decision of Jehovah's Witnesses parents to refuse blood transfusion for children under the age of 16, because such a refusal might not be in the best interests of the child (*ReS (a minor)(medical treatment)* [1993] 1 FLR 376). In making that decision, doctors have to recognise that the parents do have a right to freedom of religion, but that this must be balanced against the child's right to life (Article 2) and right to be protected from inhuman or degrading treatment (Article 3).

The refusal of treatment by an adult on the basis of religion is valid, unless the competence of that individual was questionable at the time of making the decision. Similarly, the decisions (if known) of an incompetent adult who was previously competent should be respected (e.g., unconscious Jehovah's Witnesses should not be given blood if they had refused blood transfusion when conscious).

Article 9 also respects the right of an individual to conscientiously object. Doctors, therefore, may legally claim conscientious objection to participation in abortion, withdrawal of treatment, contraception and vivisection, provided that they both refer their patients to other practitioners for care and treat patients, despite their conscientious objections, in an emergency.

**Article 10** (Freedom of Expression)

*1. Everyone has the right to freedom of expression. This right shall include the freedom to hold opinions and to receive and impart information and ideas without interference by public authority and regardless of frontiers.*

Article 10 adds to the requirement that doctors improve the quality of information given to patients, for the purpose of informing decisions or obtaining consent.

In *R v Secretary of State for Health, ex parte Wagstaff* [2000] All ER (D) 1021, the court was asked to consider whether an enquiry should take evidence in public or in private, with reference to Article 10(1). The action was brought by relatives of the deceased and Associated Newspapers Ltd, following the conviction of Dr Harold Shipman (the General Practitioner from Manchester found guilty, in January 2000, of murdering 15 of his patients). In deciding to compel the enquiry into the public arena, the court noted that, although there was no uniform practice in deciding whether an enquiry should take place in private or in public, Article 10 provided a presumption in law that an enquiry should take place in public unless there were persuasive arguments for taking another course. This decision reflects the trend towards greater openness in the conduct of enquiries following disasters (e.g. the Bristol Royal Infirmary children's cardiac surgery inquiry) and may require future enquiries by public authorities, including GMC disciplinary proceedings, to take place in public.

**Article 14** (Prohibition of Discrimination)

*The enjoyment of rights and freedoms set forth in this Convention shall be secured without discrimination on any ground such as sex, race, colour, language, religion, political or other opinion, association with a national minority, property, birth or other status.*

Article 14 is not a free standing right, but relevant in the determination of other rights. A breach of Article 14, therefore, occurs when another article has been breached and the breach has occurred in a discriminatory way. For example, the delayed provision of intensive therapy unit (ITU) care for an elderly patient, which might be held a breach of Article 3, might also be held to be a breach of Article 14, if a decision to delay treatment was affected by the patient's age. Clinical indicators demonstrating a poorer outcome for elderly patients admitted to intensive care units cannot justify blanket decisions about intensive care access. Care should be judged on individual merit. However, futile, ineffective or unproven treatment may be denied any individual, by reference to Articles 2 and 3. In a similar fashion, doctors must avoid blanket decisions relating to age when defining the resuscitation status of a patient; Articles 2 and 6 also support the notion that patients and their relatives should be involved in decisions concerning a patient's resuscitation status.

## FURTHER READING

### Books

Almond B Rights. In: Singer P (Ed). *A Companion to Ethics*. Blackwell, Oxford, 1991, pp. 259–269

Clayton R and Tomlinson H. *The Law of Human Rights*. Oxford University Press, Oxford, 2000

de Mello R (Ed). *Human Rights Act 1998. A Practical Guide*. Jordans, Bristol, 2000

Wadham J and Mountfield H (Eds). *Blackstone's Guide to the Human Rights Act*, 2nd edition. Blackstone Press, London, 1998

### Journals

Brahams D. UK: Impact of European Human Rights Law. *Lancet* 2000; **356**: 1433–1434

Hewson B. Why the human rights act matters to doctors. *Br Med J* 2000; **321**: 780–781

Horton R. Health and the UK Human Rights Act, 1998. *Lancet* 2000; **356**: 1186–1188

White SM and Baldwin TJ. The Human Rights Act, 1998: implications for anaesthesia and intensive care. *Anaesthesia* 2002; **57**: 882–888

Wicks E. The right to refuse medical treatment under the European Convention on Human Rights. *Med Law Rev* 2001; **9**: 17–40

### Internet

Human Rights Act, 1998. www.homeoffice.gov.uk/hract/guidlist.htm

*Pretty v UK*.
http://hudoc.echr.coe.int/hudoc/ViewRoot.asp?Item = 0&Action = Html&X = 1009181031&Notice = 0&Noticemode = &RelatedMode = 0

The Impact of the Human Rights Act, 1998 on Medical Decision Making. October 2000. BMA web site: http://www.bma.org.uk/public/ethics.nsf

### Legal cases

*NHS Trust A v M; NHS Trust B v H* [2001] 2 WLR 942

*The Queen on the application of Mrs Diane Pretty (Appellant) v Director of Public Prosecutions (Respondent) and Secretary of State for the Home Department (Interested Party)* [2001] UKHL 61

# 5

# Consent

Obtaining consent from a patient is not the same as having the patient sign a consent form. Instead, consent should be viewed as a legal and ethical concept that reflects the respect given by a society towards the autonomy of its citizens.

In a medical setting, consent allows an autonomous patient (i.e. one who has the capacity to think, decide and act on the basis of such thought, independently and without hindrance) to define and protect his or her own interests and to control bodily privacy. In law, consent is a device that protects the autonomy of a patient from interference by another party. Any doctor, for example, may be liable in battery or assault if (s)he administers a treatment to a patient without obtaining valid consent from them. Legal sanctions, including awards of damages, injunctions and (in extreme cases) imprisonment are employed to ensure that patient autonomy is respected.

Recourse to the law, however, does not necessarily address the thornier moral problem of *why* doctors should respect their patients' autonomy, and why they should respect it in preference to other principles that influence the relationship (such as paternalism). Nevertheless, respect for autonomy has become a central pillar of contemporary medical law and ethics, and has resulted in a greater emphasis on patient-centred determination of treatment strategies.

## ETHICS

### Autonomy

Many authors have attempted to provide an all-encompassing definition of autonomy (Greek: *autos* – 'self', *nomos* – 'rule'). Essentially, autonomy confers the idea that autonomous individuals are those capable of exercising deliberate and meaningful choices that are consistent with their own values. In other words, autonomous individuals are considered as the best judges of their own best interests.

Downie and Telfer recognised that autonomy can be displayed in one of four areas:

- *Autonomy of action*: A person is autonomous if they can choose what or what not to do, as opposed to being compelled to act or not act (i.e. they can act voluntarily).
- *Autonomy of thought*: A person is autonomous if they can choose what to think. Other authors have subsequently indicated that autonomous thoughts should be rational in nature, being consistent with a person's life goals. Rational thought demands that decisions are made on the basis of a correct understanding of the facts presented when evaluated in a logical manner, with some insight shown into the likely consequences of the decision. Note that the final determination does not have to be a *sensible* one, but just one that is in concordance with a person's life plan; for example, a fit patient with a severe compound fracture of the ankle may refuse amputation on the grounds that he 'could not live life as an amputee'.
- *Autonomy of moral judgement*: A person is autonomous if they develop their own moral belief system, and allow their actions to be determined by their beliefs, accordingly (e.g. becoming a blood donor).
- *Autonomy of moral individuality*: A person is autonomous if they can determine their own actions, independent of other influences, and should be judged by others on the basis of the subject's moral standards rather than that of societies.

Autonomy sits comfortably with the principal ethical theories described in Chapter 3. In virtue ethics, autonomy may be considered a virtue, intercedent between solipsism (total self-concern) and heteronomy (excessive passivity). However, it has been pointed out that 'a villain is surely not rendered in any way virtuous by his autonomy' (Gillon).

Deontology envisages a 'duty of respect for autonomy' in this instance, such that the duty is both a necessary part of being a rational person, *and* is required so that other persons can continue to function as rational agents.

Utilitarianism and consequentialist theory suggest that respect for autonomy maximises general happiness (although a utilitarian might also argue for the rejection of an individual's autonomy in circumstances where its recognition could increase unhappiness). Both deontology and utilitarianism recognise that there appears to be some intrinsic value in self-determination, without which individuals are vulnerable to treatment for treatment's sake, and are denied the autonomy on which much of human happiness is founded.

In medical settings, patients and physicians will usually agree about proposed treatments. However, respect for self-determination becomes problematic when conflict arises, particularly when patients reject advice that is perceived to be medically in their best interests (e.g. a patient rejecting regional anaesthesia and choosing general anaesthesia, when the latter might markedly increase their perioperative morbidity).

Proponents of patient's autonomy provide a strong argument in favour of self-determination in such an instance; in rejecting medical advice, patients may determine that the benefits and risks of treatment do not accord with their sense of self. This is a value judgement that only the patient can make, because it is the sum decision reached through the self-integration of all the abstract components of an individual's personality, components that could never be discerningly evaluated by the physician in determining the patient's overall (as opposed to merely their medical) best interests. Nevertheless, opponents might argue that patients are never fully autonomous in a medical setting, by virtue of the fact that they rely on the opinions of others in order to make a judgement concerning a proposed treatment. In addition, the patient may only be offered a limited range of medical treatments by a practitioner, which further limits their choice. Moreover, the patient may be subject to challenge or erosion of their autonomy and some form of sanction that overrides their freedom to choose if they reject a proposed course of treatment, for example sectioning under the Mental Health Act or a determination of incompetence by a doctor.

## Partial autonomy

At first sight, consent appears to enshrine a core value of contemporary medical practice, empowering patients to remain in control of their fate and bodily integrity, free from unwarranted interference from others. Indeed, it has been shown that the retention of autonomous medical decision-making capacity is associated with both improved patient satisfaction and more favourable medical outcomes. Moreover, it facilitates medical practice, and gives doctors a greater sense of value when treating patients.

However, not all patients are fully autonomous. Temporary unconsciousness is an obvious case in point. Children, for example, are autonomous in that they are capable of independent thought and deed, but the degree of autonomy they possess is not that of a competent adult. A continuum may be envisaged along which mental, physical and moral development matures towards full autonomy, but this results in applying either a status approach (i.e. autonomy above a certain age) or a functional approach (i.e. autonomy in making some decisions but not others) to autonomy. Similarly, mental illness may transiently or permanently limit personal autonomy, but again, such limitations may be circumstantial – a suicidal patient may still retain the capacity to consent to appendicectomy.

More contentiously, it could be argued that illness, fear and fear of illness themselves limit true autonomy, and to varying degrees. Again, one might envisage a continuum of severity of illness. One end of the continuum represents minor conditions that are associated with minimal effects on personal autonomy (e.g. removal of sebaceous cyst under local anaesthesia); the other end represents severe medical conditions that necessitate a dependency on medical treatment (e.g. surgical repair of a ruptured aortic aneurysm).

If patients are never more than partially autonomous (through illness, treatment or dependency on treatment), then there must be a threshold level of capacity above which the autonomy of a patient should be respected, and below which a patient is considered insufficiently autonomous to decide for themselves about treatment. The question is – who decides what this level should be? It cannot be the patient; capacity, then, must be determined by a third party (such as the perioperative physician), which involves an inevitably paternalistic process. Libertarian critics of this conclusion argue that patient autonomy should always prevail. Such critics argue that even sick patients should be allowed to assert their autonomy through consent. However, such a simplistic conclusion cannot be right. For example, the septic trauma victim who refuses anaesthesia for the surgical stabilisation of a fractured pelvis would be extremely unlikely to refuse anaesthesia if he were sufficiently 'mature in his faculties'.

A final conceptual problem involves the quantity and quality of information that is required by a patient in order to form an autonomous decision with regard to accepting or rejecting medical treatment opinion. It could be argued that if a patient is never fully in receipt of all the facts that might influence a decision about treatment, their autonomy is always compromised. Even the most rigorous research by a patient is unlikely to reveal the quantity of quality of medical information that is possessed by their doctor. Moreover, the doctor has had time to assimilate the information, rejecting that which they consider false or irrelevant and refining that which appears to be true, a process of reflection that is a function of experience, and which incorporates deliberation of all the subtle nuances of medical fact. The only way of preserving patient autonomy would be for the doctor to act as a dispassionate conduit for all facts and opinions, leaving patients to assimilate the knowledge for themselves. However, this reduces the doctor–patient relationship to one that is based on data transfer, which is clearly not why the majority of patients solicit medical advice: they are seeking both information *and specialist medical opinion*. By doing so, it could be argued that their decisions are always to some extent partially autonomous, because they involve the third-party opinions of their doctor, opinions which will be biased in favour of the patient's best medical interests.

## Paternalism

The notion of partial autonomy has two possible consequences for medical decision making. The patient is determined to be either partially self-determining in every decision (a status approach: for example whether or not to have general anaesthesia or regional anaesthesia, or both, during hernia repair), or it is decided that there are some decisions that the patient is incapable of making (a threshold approach: e.g. the surgical method of hernia repair they would prefer). In either instance, another opinion is required in order to reach the final decision. Usually, the physician offers this opinion, after an assessment of the best interests of the patient. Such beneficence is a core philosophy of medicine, and is the rationale behind medical paternalism.

Paternalism has popularly come to represent a deliberate attempt by a knowledgeable elite to limit personal rights and curb consumer choice, and is seen as the direct moral antithesis of autonomy. Indeed, paternalism from this perspective is open to legitimate criticism. The argument most commonly advanced states that doctors can never know enough about their patient's best interests to make decisions for them. Best interests are more than just medical best interests, and involve other values that are of importance to the patient, values which a doctor cannot and will not be able to ever appreciate. However, this is a theoretical barrier that exists whatever may be the philosophical position.

Another argument suggests that paternalism is open to professional abuse by inviting decisions based on medical self-interest rather than patient interest. Consider the example of the anaesthetist who prescribes regular injections of morphine to consenting National Health Service (NHS) patients after laparotomy because it is quick and effective, but persuades private patients to consent to epidural analgesia, because this attracts a larger fee for service. Critics might cite this practice as an abuse of power and an indictment of paternalism. Here the anaesthetist has acted in their self-interest before patient interest in both instances. However, such practices are more a representation of a flaw of character and integrity of the doctor rather than a flaw of paternalism. It is arguable that such flaws are best dealt with by a robust response from a medical disciplinary committee rather than by wrongly attributing this flaw to be a result of a vital component of medical paternalism.

The most divisive argument concerns whether beneficence is of greater moral importance than respect for autonomy. Both utilitarianism and deontology can accommodate paternalism. Paternalism has utilitarian moral worth if it maximises welfare, and can only be subordinated by autonomy if the consequences of paternalism produce less happiness than autonomous action (or if autonomy is viewed as an independent determinant of happiness). Paternalism sits less well in deontology, because it tends to advocate the use of people as means to an end. However, the practice of medicine is fundamentally deontological in nature – 'do no harm' and 'act in the patients' best interests' are the common tenets and ethical principles. Respect for autonomy is merely one of a number of duties that the doctor should strive to follow (as part of 'pluralist' deontology). Whether the doctor respects patient autonomy ahead of paternalistic action, or vice-versa, depends on which of the competing duties is the most compelling. Current medical thinking makes respect for autonomy more of an imperative than benevolent paternalism, the converse only being permitted if a patient clearly lacks autonomy, or explicitly entrusts their best interests to the doctor. In the first instance, consent may be impossible to obtain (e.g. when faced with an unconscious patient). In the second, the patient may tell the doctor to do 'what they think is best', or implicitly entrust their welfare to the doctor by, for example, signing a consent form without reading it.

Nevertheless, there are a number of instances in perioperative medicine and critical care in which paternalism may be justified. Firstly, the welfare of the patient may be served best by paternalistic intervention. In cases involving severe injury or unconsciousness, the doctor might reasonably expect that the patient would consent to intervention were (s)he conscious or fully competent ('predictive' consent). Not only are there potentially life-saving benefits for the patient, but there is no loss of autonomy, because the patient is unable to consent, and there is no reason to suppose the patient would object. Intervention would be justified, for example, if the patient verbally refused treatment (e.g. suturing lacerations in inebriated patients), or in order to return a patient to normal health (e.g. intubating a patient with facial injuries resulting from a car accident), or to prevent further deterioration in their condition (e.g. intubating a conscious, severe asthmatic who is unable to speak).

Secondly, patients may waive their autonomy. If the patient refuses to entertain any information about the intervention proposed, any consent given would be invalid. Nevertheless, waivers should be treated with scepticism, particularly when apparently subject to denial or fear (common emotions amongst patients, perioperatively). However, should the patient waive their autonomy because they feel unfamiliar with the decision-making process, are badly informed, or think that their doctor knows best, there is an onus on the doctor to seek their consent. The information given to such patients may be more paternalistic in nature, because what the patients seemingly require in this instance is opinion rather than sufficient information on which to form their own, independent decisions.

Thirdly, degrees of paternalism may be justified according to individual patient competence. The benefit may be absolute (if the patient has never been competent or is unlikely to return to a state of adequate competence) or relative, enabling either a return to health (e.g. intensive care) or continued health until a level of competence is reached (e.g. paediatric surgery). A sliding scale of risk-dependent, functional competence that justifies compensatory paternalism has been proposed by some authors, but rejected by others who argue for a status approach (the patient is either competent or not, greater risk requiring a more intense assessment of competence).

Finally, the patient may just make 'bad' decisions. Pro-autonomists might argue that a patient never makes a bad decision, merely one that contrasts drastically with the doctor's opinions. It must be that this assertion is wrong. For example, a competent patient may decide after receiving relevant information that he does not wish to receive any analgesia after a major bowel operation, because all methods of analgesia proposed have side-effects. This decision is autonomous, but undoubtedly a poor one for the patient, and to an extent may justify coercive attempts by the doctor to get the patient to change their mind.

Savulescu has noted that 'patients can fail to make correct judgements of what is best, just as doctors can'. Savulescu argues that patients do this by failing to make choices that best satisfy their own values (e.g. refusing postoperative analgesia), or by making choices that frustrate rather than facilitate their autonomy (e.g. accepting the need for general anaesthesia during major surgery, but refusing intravenous cannulation), or by making incorrect value judgements (i.e. failing to attach the appropriate significance to the relevant facts when making a decision). In these situations, further discussion with the patient may reveal reasons behind their 'poor' judgement, and the provision of additional information may resolve any contention between both parties.

Nevertheless, there will be instances when the doctor may continue to believe that a degree of coercion is warranted. Consider the case of a patient, Mr A, who is due to undergo surgical repair of a 10 cm abdominal aortic aneurysm, but who refuses intraoperative blood transfusion, because he is worried of the infinitesimally small risk of contracting variant Jakob–Creutzfeld disease (vCJD) through transfusion. Mr A's anaesthetist may explore these fears in a preoperative visit, and may discuss alternative methods of fluid replacement or conservation during this potentially very bloody operation. However, if the patient still refuses blood transfusion, the anaesthetist is faced with a conundrum – it would be morally and professionally very difficult to justify proceeding without potential recourse to transfusion, because of the markedly greater risk of severe patient morbidity or mortality. This example differs from the problems posed by blood-refusing Jehovah's Witnesses, in that such patients refuse blood based on a strongly held religious belief, a belief that forms a core value to them, and is therefore to be respected. Mr A, however, although making an apparently autonomous decision about an admittedly possible but realistically negligible risk is undoubtedly making a poor decision, one that may be viewed as being at odds with his normal beliefs and values. The easiest course for the anaesthetist is just to respect Mr A's decision, and proceed. Alternatively, the anaesthetist may respect Mr A's refusal, but then refuse to anaesthetise Mr A because of the substantially increased perioperative risk to him. Nevertheless, this course of conduct may compromise a duty to treat Mr A. However, hard cases make for hard decisions. In these circumstances it is arguable that the anaesthetist may be justified in coercing Mr A into accepting blood. If left untreated, a 10 cm aneurysm would be likely to rupture within a year, with a 90% mortality if this occurred outside hospital, an occurrence that the anaesthetist may decide does not conform with Mr A's values (Mr A being an otherwise happy family man). The anaesthetist may feel that Mr A has attached undue weight to the risk of vCJD, and may continue to try and convince Mr A to accept blood.

This problem raises the question as to whether there are limits to the extent to which doctors should attempt to coerce patients into accepting their advice? Certainly – although it is a fine (and often indistinct) line between *coercing* a patient to accept treatment (which maintains or enhances their autonomy), and *compelling* them to accept treatment (which erodes their autonomy). Savulescu's concept of 'rational, non-interventional paternalism' acknowledges this, that the anaesthetist should make a value judgement of what is best for the patient. This fulfils his/her duty as a moral agent, and may benefit patient autonomy through rational presentation of treatment options, but rejects the use of compulsion in the therapeutic relationship (i.e. is 'non-interventional').

## Trust

Both autonomy and paternalism have practical and philosophical limitations. Why, then, has society sought to promote the principle of respect for autonomy at the expense of medical paternalism?

Traditionally, the doctor–patient relationship consisted of a paternalistic association based on trust. Patients trusted their doctors advice because they had no other sources of information, respected the knowledge that doctors possessed and believed that their doctor was always acting in their best interests. However, this situation has changed. Today patients are much better informed about their condition, the advance of technology has outstripped many doctors' ability to keep pace with change, 'quality assurance' initiatives provide league tables of doctors, which are available for public scrutiny, and medical litigation promotes unconditional respect for patient autonomy whilst exposing medical 'errors'.

Although the changes have for the most part been welcomed by the medical profession, they have undoubtedly led to an erosion of trust between patients and doctors, such that consent has been transformed from a mechanism of doctor–patient communication into a defensive legal instrument that hinders respect for patient autonomy. Consent has effectively *replaced* trust as the basis for doctor–patient relationships. However, this should not be viewed as the victory of autonomy over paternalism: rather that the loss of trust in the doctor–patient relationship has been replaced by patients' self-determination of where to place their trust. Patients may trust their own judgement based on assessments of information acquired, or may request further information from doctors and choose whether to accept the advice or not. This choice places a greater responsibility for decision-making on the patient, but is lessened if there is trust between patient and doctor, such that the patient readily accepts the advice given and the doctor conveys trustworthy information. Consent in a trusting relationship maximises patient welfare by respecting *both* patient autonomy and medical beneficence.

## LAW

In law, 'informed consent' is an instrument that engenders respect for autonomy. In the medical setting, informed consent allows an individual to define and protect his or her own interests and to control bodily privacy. A doctor may be liable in the tort or crime of battery if (s)he administers treatment to a patient without their consent. Retaining the capacity to make autonomous medical decisions has been shown both to improve patient satisfaction, and medical outcomes.

However, there are a number of instances in which patients' decision-making capacity is compromised. Some, such as unconsciousness and dementia are obvious. The majority of cases are less clear, and relate to degrees of partial autonomy – children, the mentally ill or even those with illness *per se* may be capable of independent thought and deed, but may not be judged to possess sufficient legal capacity to give consent.

Consent may be expressed or implied, the form in which it is given having no bearing on its validity. Consent may be implied from the conduct of the patient. For example, consent might be implied, when the patient holds out their arm to the doctor for an injection, rather than giving an express verbal agreement. Expressed consent may take the form of a verbal assent or written agreement, although a signed consent form merely acts as documentary evidence, rather than the legal affirmation, of valid consent – this is important: consent is not about getting the patient to sign a consent form!

Consent may be withdrawn at any point. Withdrawal of consent renders subsequent treatment unlawful.

Consent is legally valid if it is given **voluntarily** by an **appropriately informed** person, who has the requisite **capacity** to exercise an informed choice.

## Voluntariness

Voluntariness may be affected by a number of perioperative circumstances, including the nature of the patient's disease, the range of treatment therapies offered, family and religious considerations, and the doctor–patient dynamic. The problem of whether consent is voluntarily given may be further complicated in instances where the patient is a prisoner, or detainee of a psychiatric hospital.

A leading English case is that of *Re T (adult: refusal of treatment)* [1992] 4 All ER 649, in which the Court of Appeal upheld the lower courts decision to allow the transfusion of blood to a critically ill Jehovah's Witness, on the basis that the patient had refused transfusion on religious grounds after undue persuasion by her mother.

## Capacity

In the conclusion of her judgement in *Re MB (an adult: medical treatment)* [1997] 38 BMLR 175 (CA) (in which a mother consented to Caesarian section at term for breech presentation of her baby, but not intravenous cannulation – her refusal was overruled), Dame Elizabeth Butler-Sloss stated:

'Every person is presumed to have the capacity to consent to or refuse medical treatment unless and until that presumption is rebutted'

and that:

'a person lacks capacity if some impairment or disturbance of mental function renders the person unable to make a decision whether to consent to, or refuse, treatment. That inability to make a decision will occur when:
– the patient is unable to *comprehend and retain the information* which is material to the decision, especially as to the likely consequences of having, or not having, the treatment in question;
– the patient is unable to *use the information and weigh it in the balance* as part of the process of arriving at the decision'.

Therefore, valid consent requires that the perioperative physician make a judgement of a patient's capacity to make an informed choice concerning medical intervention.

Several issues need to be emphasised. First, the decision made by the patient does not have to be sensible, rational or well considered. Although consent/refusal made on the basis of an irrational belief which is contrary to the evidence and not widely held by society might indicate that the patient is suffering from mental illness (*St Georges NHS Trust v S* [1998] 3 All ER 673 (CA)). Where a patient's competence is in doubt, declaratory relief should be sought from the courts.

Secondly, the more serious the decision to be made, the proportionately greater the level of capacity is required (*ReT(adult: refusal of treatment)* [1992] 4 All ER 649).

Thirdly, contemporaneous competent *refusals* of treatment carry the same legal force as a competently given consent (*ReT(adult: refusal of treatment)* [1992] 4 All ER 649).

Finally, in the case of adults no other person (including the courts or those with legal powers of attorney) may consent to medical treatment for an incapacitated (or other) adult. However, the courts have stated that doctors have a legal duty however to treat incompetent patients in accordance with the concept of *best interests*, which necessitates wider assessment of the patient's welfare than what the benefits of medical treatment might be (*ReF (mental patient: sterilisation)* [1990] 2 AC 1 (HL)).

## Information

A number of clinical studies have been performed in order to assess what patients would like to know about their treatment. The results of these studies did not reveal a simple answer. Many patients prefer to be given simple descriptions of procedures and explanation about the main risks and benefits, although a significant number would like to receive full information about procedures and risks.

In order to defend an action in battery (battery is the intentional touching, however slight, of another's person without their consent), a doctor must be able to provide sufficient evidence that (s)he supplied the patient with adequate information about the *nature and purpose* of the procedure (i.e. a doctor has committed a battery even if the patient has consented, if the doctor cannot prove that (s)he told the patient why he was touching them). Although the legal burden proof of lack of consent remains with the victim/claimant/patient the evidential burden of proof in battery lies with the toucher (doctor/nurse/etc.) (i.e. they need to provide documentary or other evidence that the patient consented). An action in the tort of battery is actionable *per se* such that the victim does not have to demonstrate that they suffered any physical or mental harm as a result of the touching but merely they were touched without consent.

In order to pursue an action in negligence, the plaintiff must prove, among other things, both that the doctor failed to disclose information about the *risks and consequences* of the procedure, and that but for the negligent failure to advise, the patient would have declined treatment (i.e. the doctor is negligent if the patient can prove that the doctor did not inform them of possible outcomes of treatment). Note that the burden of proof in negligence is on the touched (i.e. the patient).

The legal position with regard to information disclosure in the United Kingdom has moved from the 'reasonable doctor' standard of *Bolam* towards the 'reasonable patient' standard suggested by Lord Scarman in *Sidaway*. After *Bolam*, (*Bolam v Friern Barnet Hospital Management Committee* [1957] 1 WLR 582), the doctor only needed to disclose that which a responsible body of medical practitioners might disclose. The standard of care was determined as that 'of the ordinary skilled man exercising and professing to have that special skill'; the doctor was not negligent if he acted in accordance with a practice accepted at the time as proper by a responsible body of medical opinion, even if other doctors accepted different practices.

After *Sidaway* (*Sidaway v Board of Governors of Bethlem Royal Hospital and the Maudsley Hospital* [1985] 1 AC 871), however, doctors have a duty to warn a patient about a material risk if 'the court is satisfied that a reasonable person in the patient's position would be likely to attach significance to the risk', unless 'he takes the view that a warning would be detrimental to his patient's health'. This approach was confirmed in *Pearce* (*Pearce v United Bristol Healthcare NHS Trust* [1998] 48 BMLR 118

(CA)), in which it was judged that there was a duty to disclose information that the patient would consider significant, the standard of the information being decided by the *court* rather than the doctors. Decisions to withhold information by doctors (on the grounds of the information being detrimental to the patient's health – a form of 'therapeutic privilege') are only sanctioned by the court if they are rational, responsible and responsive. The legal burden of demonstrating a therapeutic necessity lies with the doctor.

The main problem that arises with all the above case law concerns the definition of 'significant risk'. The law equates significant material risk with a degree of risk to which a patient would attach relevance. However, different patients on different occasions will interpret risk differently. The interpretation of material risk will always be inconsistent. The problem for doctors in general is that scientific risk equates to a numerical value, but the courts have been reluctant thus far to define what such an incidence might be in terms of 'significant' risk. Every medical procedure performed carries a range of risks, which may be minor or major in consequence, common or rare in incidence, causal or incidental to the harm sustained (if any), convenient or inconvenient in timing, expected or unexpected, relative or absolute, operator dependent or any combination of the above. In addition, there are significant difficulties in communicating risk, caused by patient perceptions, anaesthetist perceptions and the doctor–patient interaction, and complicated by the range of communication methods (numerical (percent/incidence/logarithmic/degree scale), verbal or descriptive).

Professional bodies have attempted to address the obscurity of the legal definition of significant risk by publishing guidelines detailing what doctors should disclose to their patients. However, these tend merely to restate the legal position. Whilst providing examples of the type of risks and consequences that might be disclosed; the onus is still very much on the doctor to pitch the level of disclosure according to the rather abstract concept of 'what a reasonable patient would consider significant'. The only way to overcome this problem would be to fully disclose all risks and consequences. However, this is likely to bewilder and alarm the majority of patients, and could lead to situations in which patients consent to one treatment, for example, to blood transfusion, but refuse an ancillary procedure, such as intravenous access.

In future, there may be a duty to disclose alternatives to the proposed treatment, or to advise the patient about non-treatment or the consequences of non-treatment.

Figure 5.1 summarises the process of determining consent to medical treatment by adult patients.

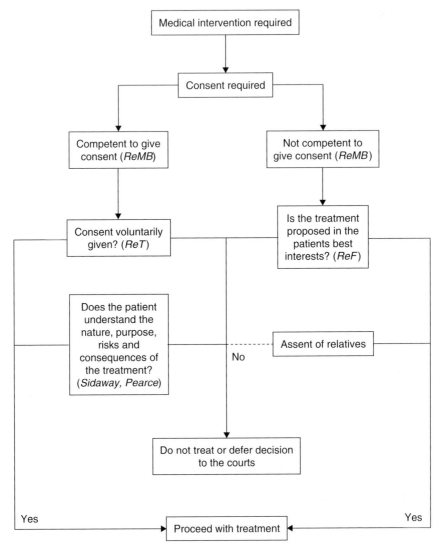

**Figure 5.1** Consent pathway for adults.

## Refusal of treatment

Similarly to consent for treatment, adults may refuse any and every treatment if they are competent and informed, and make the decision voluntarily, even if this will result in their death (*B v An NHS Trust* [2002] EWHC 429 (Fam)). Refusal of treatment that results in death is not considered a form of suicide.

However, the right to refuse medical treatment might be overruled by the courts in the public interest (e.g. preserving the life of innocent third parties, preventing suicide or homicide, and preserving the professional integrity of doctors). Nevertheless, English law has not, as yet, gone this far and at present third party interests are considered irrelevant for the purposes of the law (see *ReMB*).

Advance refusals of treatment are considered in detail in Chapter 11.

## 'Incompetents'

Perioperative physicians are likely to encounter a number of patients whose capacity and volition are affected either by their age or their medical condition. The following 'special circumstances' address the application of English common law to such patients.

### *Children*

Under Section 8(1)–(3) of the Family Law Reform Act, 1969, 16- and 17-year- old children are *rebuttably presumed to be competent* to give consent for any surgical, medical or dental treatment that would otherwise constitute a battery on them (*ReW (a minor)(medical treatment)* [1993] Fam 64 (CA)). Therefore, 16- and 17-year olds are presumed competent to consent unless it can be shown that they are incompetent, such that they fail the two stage test of competence stated in *ReMB* (the patient is competent if they can take in and retain information, use it and weigh it in the balance). However, it should be noted that both Section 8(1) of the Family Law Reform Act, 1969, *ReR* and *ReW* discuss *consent* to treatment. *Refusals* of treatment by competent 16- and 17-year olds are likely to be overruled by the court.

Children under the age of 16 are *rebuttably presumed to be incompetent* to consent to treatment (although this is not the case in Scotland – under Section 2(4) of the Age of Legal Capacity (Scotland) Act, 1991 a 'person under the age of 16 years shall have legal capacity to consent on his own behalf to any surgical, medical or dental procedure or treatment where, in the opinion of a qualified medical practitioner attending him, he is capable of understanding the nature and possible consequences of the procedure or treatment'). However, a *Gillick* competent child can consent to treatment (*Gillick v West Norfolk and Wisbech Area Health Authority*), their competence being a question of fact, such that the child can give valid consent if they can understand the nature and implications of the proposed treatment. *Gillick* competent under 16s should be encouraged to inform their parents about treatment, but a refusal to do so forbids the doctor from disclosure to the parents. When the consequences of a decision puts the child's life at risk, a very high level of understanding may be required by the court – the courts have proved very adverse to any child refusing potentially life-saving medical treatment, overruling their refusals even if they legally competent. However, English law has yet to consider a case in light of either the United Nations Convention on the Rights of the Child or the Human Rights Act, 1998 (specifically Articles 3 and 8).

*Proxy consent* may be provided for incompetent children by parents, temporary carers, local authorities or the courts, provided the consent is given in the best interests of the patient (which are not necessarily the medical best interests). Parents (or those with parental responsibility according to the Children Act, 1989 namely legal guardians nominated by the parents, unmarried fathers who have entered and registered a parental rights agreement) are the most obvious repositories of proxy decision-making power, though they themselves must be competent to make the decision and it must be made in the child's best interests. Each parent has the right to consent (Section 2(7) of the Children Act, 1989, Article 8 of the Human Rights Act, 1998), though when a major decision has to be made there may be a duty incumbent on the consenting parent to inform the other parent. If there is disagreement between the parents, the courts may limit the power of one parent to refuse treatment that is in the best interests of the child. If both parents refuse, an application may be made to the court to overrule the parents.

Temporary carers include teachers and doctors. Anyone over 16 who has responsibility for a child under 16 has a duty to obtain essential medical assistance for the child (Section 1 Children and Young Persons Act, 1933). Likewise, anyone who does not have parental responsibility but has care of a child may do all that is reasonable to secure the welfare of the child (Section 3(5) Children Act, 1989). Although it is usually not lawful to do so, doctors may treat children without any proxy consent if it is impossible/impractical to seek consent from a parent or the court under the doctrine of necessity. Alternatively, if the parents refuse and the treatment is vital and there is no time to seek the court's assent to the treatment.

A local authority which has care of a child has parental responsibility (Section 33(3)(a) Children Act, 1989) and can therefore make treatment decisions. The courts may provide proxy consent in one of three ways: by making the child a ward of court, by employing its inherent jurisdiction, or by making a specific issue or a prohibited steps order.

Figure 5.2 summarises the process of determining consent to medical treatment by patients under the age of 18 years.

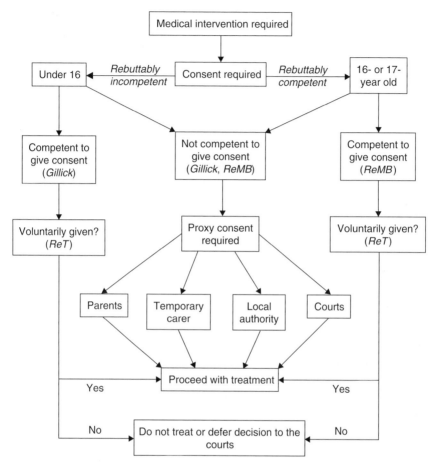

**Figure 5.2** Consent pathway for under Section 18 (England).

## Mental illness and the Mental Health Act, 1983

Mental illness may impair a patient's capacity to provide valid consent or refusal for an anaesthetic intervention. However, a person receiving treatment for mental illness should not be assumed to be incapable of providing valid consent for treatment (*ReC (adult: refusal of medical treatment)* [1994] 1 All ER 819). In English law, it is clear that no one may consent to medical treatment on behalf of a mentally incompetent adult. Non-consensual medical treatment is therefore only possible on the grounds of necessity and in the best interests of the patient.

Part IV of the Mental Health Act, 1983 (MHA) deals with issues of consent and non-consensual treatment for those with a defined mental illness (amongst many other things). Section 63 states that 'the consent of a patient shall not be required for any medical treatment given to him *for the mental disorder from which he is suffering*' – that is consent is still required for treatment that is not aimed at curing his medical condition. Even then, the patient's consent is still required for:

- psychosurgery (requires consent and a second opinion, Section 57);
- electroconvulsive therapy (ECT) (requires consent or a second opinion, Section 58).

The MHA has recently been extensively reviewed in the White Paper *Reforming the Mental Health Act*, Chapter 5 of which deals with criteria for compulsory care and treatment, and Chapter 9 of which deals with treatment. Psychosurgery still requires patient consent and a second opinion. Treatment proposed under Section 58 of the 1983 Act (including ECT) will be subject to special safeguards: the consent of the patient is required, or, in the case of the incapacitated, the authorisation of a mental health tribunal (rather than a second medical opinion) will be required.

## Mental incapacity bill

At the time of writing the government is intending to introduce a new statute, the Mental Incapacity Act, to England and Wales. In essence, the Act will delineate the circumstances whereby substituted decision-making ability may be employed on behalf of individuals whose capacity may be affected by 'an impairment of or disturbance in the functioning of the brain or mind'. Although the present MHA and the proposed Mental Health Bill deal with very similar issues, the concept of making a decision on behalf of another person under the new Bill is extended to include medical treatment, as well as psychiatric treatment. Two important principles will affect the practice of perioperative medicine:

- there will be a 'general authority' to treat the incompetent for medical problems, using the principle of best interests. This is a formalisation of the current common law. The general authority will makes it lawful to act for someone who lacks capacity where it is reasonable for the person taking the action to do so and the act is in the person's best interests;
- the Bill will propose a new system of Lasting Powers of Attorney (LPA), which allow people to appoint an attorney to act on their behalf if they should lose capacity in the future (Clauses 8–13, 21+22). A LPA will be applicable to welfare (including healthcare) matters as well as financial matters.

## Pregnancy

Pregnancy is a natural process for which medical intervention may be required, either throughout its duration or during labour. A number of legal issues arise. Firstly, pregnant women are no less autonomous that non-pregnant women. Pain and distress do not necessarily make a labouring woman incompetent. However, a number of decisions in the late 1990s held that labouring women were incapable of making decisions whilst in labour, which allowed the courts to authorise Caesarian sections in the best interests of the mother. This alarmed a number of agencies, who saw that health authorities and trusts were beginning to rely on the coercive threat of court intervention in order to achieve a successful delivery, despite legal assurance that competent women are allowed to refuse treatment even if this harms their foetus. Fears were calmed by Dame Elizabeth Butler-Sloss in *ReMB*, concerning the 'temporary factors' mentioned by Lord Donaldson MR in *ReT*; although confusion, shock, fatigue, pain or drugs *may* completely erode capacity, those concerned must be satisfied '*that such factors are operating to such a degree that the ability to decide is absent*'.

Birth plans should be treated as advanced directives. The legal validity of anticipatory decisions was confirmed recently in *ReAK* (*ReAK (Adult patient)(Medical treatment: consent)* [2001] 1 FLR 129). Such decisions are valid if at the time they were made the patient was informed, competent and made the decision voluntarily, and the decision was intended to apply in the circumstances arising.

## Emergencies

Emergency medical treatment excludes the requirement for informed consent. There may even be duty to provide medical treatment, provided the treatment is both necessary and cannot be reasonably delayed. This holds for adults, children and the otherwise incompetent.

## Teaching

It is incumbent on medical students (or other students) themselves, rather than their medical teachers, to seek consent from patients **before** examining patients. This includes examinations under anaesthesia. Students must make it clear that they are students, and should avoid the fraudulent assertion that they are qualified medical professionals. Not to do so exposes the student to liability in battery and negligence.

Similarly, consent must be obtained prior to taking photographs or video recordings of the patient. Consent must also be obtained before retaining tissue for teaching purposes.

## Additional procedures

If it becomes obvious during surgery on an anaesthetised patient that a further procedure is needed for which consent has not been obtained, then the surgeon may proceed without consent provided that the extra intervention is necessary and in the patient's best interests (e.g. a life-saving splenectomy during emergency surgery for blunt abdominal trauma), unless that extra procedure has been explicitly forbidden by the patient preoperatively when competent.

## Jehovah's Witnesses

There are approximately 6 million Jehovah's Witnesses worldwide, with an estimated 150,000 resident in the UK.

In 1945, the spiritual administration of the Jehovah's Witnesses decided that followers should not receive transfused blood or blood products, based on several passages in the Bible (Genesis 9: 3–4, Leviticus 17: 11–12 and Acts 15: 28–29). Although there is variation amongst adherents in the strength of this belief, those with the greatest depth of faith refuse blood (or blood product) transfusion, even if this could lead to personal harm or death, believing that to receive a transfusion will result in their eternal damnation. Organ transplantation is not expressly forbidden, and is a matter of personal choice (as is auto-transfusion, if provided in a closed circuit, and acceptance of fractionated blood products, such as immunoglobulins).

Jehovah's Witnesses are generally well informed about their legal position. Most carry an advanced directive card (see Chapter 12), and have contacted their general practitioner and local hospitals with regard their faith and wishes in the event of treatment. Provided that their advanced directive was made voluntarily, and the patient was competent and informed when the decision was made, unauthorised blood transfusion would constitute a battery. In an emergency, doctors may administer a blood transfusion only if they are ignorant of any evidence that the patient would ordinarily have refused blood transfusion.

Courts in the UK have been reluctant to martyr the children of Jehovah's Witnesses to the parents beliefs, even if the child is deemed competent to consent to treatment (*ReS (a minor) (consent to medical treatment)* [1994] 2 FLR 1065). In practice, where there is conflict between the doctor and the parents before elective procedures, a Specific Issue Order should be sought from the Courts, authorising a blood transfusion. In an emergency, and where the child's life is in immediate danger, the doctor may administer blood without prior application to the courts.

## PRACTICAL SUMMARY OF CONSENT

- Obtaining consent from a patient is not the same as having the patient sign a consent form.
- Obtaining consent should be considered a fluid, reciprocal and patient-centred process, that empowers patient autonomy.
- A signed consent form merely acts as documentary evidence, rather than the legal affirmation, of valid consent.
- Expressed consent should be obtained for any procedure which carries a material risk (i.e. a risk to which a reasonable patient in the patient's position would be likely to attach significance).
- The clinician providing the treatment is responsible for obtaining consent from the patient.
- Valid consent can only be given by a *competent, informed* patient who assents *voluntarily* to the proposed treatment.
- Competent patients *comprehend and retain the information* which is material to their decision, and *use the information and weigh it in the balance* as part of the process of arriving at their decision.
- Information should be given as to the *nature and purpose* of treatment, in order to avoid committing a battery.
- Information should be given as to the *risks and consequences* of treatment, in order to defend actions in negligence.
- A competent adult may refuse any and all treatment, even if it is life-saving.
- *Incompetent adults*: No other person can consent to or refuse treatment on behalf of an incompetent adult. However, treatment may proceed or be terminated if, in the doctors' estimation, it in the best interests (though not necessarily medical best interests) of the patient. Relatives and friends should be encouraged to assent to treatment that is in the patient's best interests.
- *Children*: 16 and 17 year olds may consent to treatment, unless it can be shown that they lack the competence to do so. Under 16s may consent to treatment if they are deemed *Gillick* competent. Refusals of treatment by anyone under 18 years old may be challenged.
- Pain, distress and illness do not necessarily render a person incompetent to give consent.
- All patients should be given the opportunity to ask questions as part of the consent process, and honest answers should be provided.
- Patients detained under certain sections of the Mental Health Act, 1983, are not necessarily excluded from making medical treatment decisions.

## FURTHER READING

### Books

British Medical Association and The Law Society. *Assessment of Mental Capacity*, Guidance for doctors and lawyers. BMA Professional Division Publications, London, 2004

Department of Health. Medical students in hospitals: a guide on their access to patients and clinical work. London, Department of Health, 1997

Gillon R. Autonomy and the principle of respect for autonomy. In: *Philosophical Medical Ethics*, John Wiley and Sons, Chichester, 2000, pp. 60–72

Kennedy and Grubb (Eds). Medical Law 3rd edition. Chapter 5 and 6. Consent, and Consent by Others, pp. 575–989

Mason and McCall Smith (Eds). Law and Medical Ethics 5th edition. Chapter 10. Consent to treatment, pp. 244–288

Young R. Informed consent and patient autonomy. In: Kuhse H, Singer P (Eds). *A Companion To Bioethics*, Blackwell, Massuchusetts, 1998. pp. 441

### Journals

Adams AM and Smith AF. Risk perception and communication: recent developments and implications for anaesthesia. *Anaesthesia* 2001; **56**: 745–755

Alldridge P. Consent to medical and surgical treatment-the law commission's recommendations. *Med Law Rev* 1996; **4**: 129–143

Calman KC. Communication of risk: choice, consent and trust. *Lancet* 2002; **360**: 166–168

Commentary. Competent adult patient: right to refuse life-sustaining treatment *Re B (Adult: Refusal Of Medical Treatment). Med Law Rev* 2002; **10**: 201–204

Downie RS and Telfer E. Autonomy. *Philosophy* 1971; **178**: 293–301

Dawes PJ and Davison P. Informed consent: what do patients want to know? *J Roy Soc Med* 1994; **87**: 149–152

Habiba M. Examining consent within the patient–doctor relationship. *J Med Ethic* 2000; **26**: 183–187

Jones MA. Informed consent and other fairy stories. *Med Law Rev* 1999; **7**: 103

Jenkins K and Baker AB. Consent and anaesthetic risk. *Anaesthesia* 2003; **58**: 962–984

Lockwood GM. Pregnancy, autonomy and paternalism. *J Med Ethic* 1999; **25**: 537–540

O'Neill O. Paternalism and partial autonomy. *J Med Ethic* 1984; **10**: 173–178

Savulescu J. Rational non-interventional paternalism: why doctors ought to make judgements of what is best for their patients. *J Med Ethic* 1995; **21**: 327–331

Slovenko R. Informed consent: information about the physician. *Medicine and Law* 1994; **13**: 467–472

White SM and Baldwin TJ. Consent for anaesthesia. *Anaesthesia* 2003; **58**: 760–774

## Internet

Association of Anaesthetists of Great Britain and Ireland. Information and consent for anaesthesia, 1999. http://www.aagbi.org/pdf/consent1.pdf

British medical association. Report of the consent working party. March, 2001. www.bma.org.uk/ap.nsf/Content/report+of+the+consent+working+party

Draft mental incapacity bill. June, 2003. http://www.dca.gov.uk/menincap/overview.htm#part4

Department of Health. Reference guide to consent for examination or treatment. 2001. http://www.doh.gov.uk/consent/refguide.htm

Department of Health. Reforming the mental health act. www.doh.gov.uk/mentalhealth/whitepaper2000.htm

General Medical Council. Seeking patients' consent: the ethical considerations. 1998. http://www.gmc-uk.org/standards/consent.htm

Lord Chancellor's Department. Making decisions: Helping people who have difficulty deciding for themselves. May, 2003. http://www.lcd.gov.uk/consult/family/decisionresp.htm#part7c

Management of anaesthesia for Jehovah's Witnesses. Association of Anaesthetists of Great Britain and Ireland. March, 1999. http://www.aagbi.org/pdf/7doc.pdf

The Law Commission. Mental incapacity. Law Commission report 231. http://www.lawcom.gov.uk/library/lc231/contents.htm

## Legal cases

*Chester v Afshar* [2002] EWCA Civ 724 (CA)

*Gillick v West Norfolk and Wisbech Area Health Authority* [1986] AC 112 (HL)

*ReC (adult: refusal of medical treatment)* [1994] 1 All ER 819 (Fam Div)

*ReMB (an adult: medical treatment)* [1997] 2 FLR 426 (CA)

*ReT (adult: refusal of medical treatment)* [1992] 9 BMLR 46 (CA)

*ReF (mental patient: sterilisation)* [1990] 2 AC 1 (HL)

*ReAK (Adult patient)(Medical treatment: consent)* [2001] 1 FLR 129

*ReR (a minor)(wardship: consent to treatment)* [1992] Fam 11

*ReW (a minor)(medical treatment)* [1992] 4 All ER 627

*Sidaway v Board of Governors of Bethlem Royal Hospital and the Maudsley Hospital* [1985] 1 AC 871

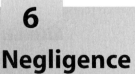

# 6
# Negligence

*'Errare humanum est'*

– attributed to Plutarch

*'Whatever houses I may visit, I will come for the benefit of the sick, remaining free of all intentional injustice, of all mischief …'*

– Hippocratic Oath

One of the most noticeable changes in medico-legal practice over the last 20 years has been the vast increase in the number of complaints from patients and their relatives. There may be a number of reasons for this, including:

- clinicians may be making more errors;
- patient expectations are higher;
- patients are more likely to sue clinicians;
- lawyers are more likely to pursue legal claims against clinicians;
- significant financial payouts act as incentives to pursue legal claims.

The cost to the National Health Service (NHS) of settled and outstanding negligence claims is enormous. Various estimates have been made. Fenn *et al.* estimated that the rate of closed claims rose by 7% per annum throughout the 1990s, and cost the NHS between £48 million and £130 million in 1998 alone. By extrapolation, the liability for claims that are yet to be settled amounts to £1.8 billion.

The gradual realisation of the cost of negligence claims to the NHS has prompted the formation of a number of bodies, in order to try and improve the safety and quality of healthcare. These include:

- The National Patient Safety Agency (NPSA). The NPSA is a Special Health Authority created in July 2001 to co-ordinate the mandatory reporting of errors and near-misses in clinical practice, with the aim of learning from mistakes and problems that affect patient safety. Importantly, staff are encouraged to report incidents without fear of personal reprimand.

- The Commission for Healthcare Audit and Inspection (CHAI) (aka the Healthcare Commission). This body was created on the 1 April (!) 2004, and is an amalgamation of Commission for Health Improvement (CHI), the National Care Standards Commission (NCSC) and those elements of the Audit Commission's work that related to the efficiency, effectiveness and economy of healthcare. The overall aim of the Healthcare Commission is to promote an improvement of the quality of NHS, private and voluntary healthcare nationwide.
- The National Clinical Assessment Authority (NCAA). The NCAA is a special health authority which aims to provide a support service to health authorities, primary care trusts and hospital and community trusts, who are faced with concerns over the performance of individual doctors and dentists.

This chapter outlines the potential causes of medical error, and the ethics behind the legal position on negligence, before providing a comprehensive review of how the law relating to negligence is applied in the UK.

## ETHICS

A large number of medical errors occur each year. Indeed, medical errors, accounting for between 44,000 and 96,000 deaths per annum, are the fourth commonest cause of death in the USA (according to Lucien Leape, the doyen of research into medical error). Approximately 4–10% of hospital inpatients suffer significant iatrogenic injury, costing an estimated £2 billion per annum in extended inpatient care; 1.7 mistakes a day are made in the treatment of intensive care patients.

### Errors, mistakes, accidents and negligence

An error occurs either when there is a failure of a planned action to be completed as intended, or when a wrong plan has been used to achieve an aim. Errors are not planned, or expected, or wanted. Errors do not necessarily result in an adverse outcome.

An adverse outcome may occur without an error having occurred (an 'undesirable outcome'), provided the intention was correct, the action was executed correctly, and the outcome was probabilistic in nature (i.e. had the potential, albeit small, to go wrong).

An adverse event is an injury caused by medical management rather than an underlying condition of the patient. An adverse event attributable to error is known as a 'preventable adverse event'.

Negligent adverse events represent a subset of preventable adverse events that satisfy the legal criteria of negligence (i.e. that harm was caused to a patient due to the clinician failing to provide an acceptable standard of medical care).

An accident is an unplanned, unexpected or undesired event that usually has an adverse outcome.

## The classification of medical error

A number of classifications have been used, according to the interaction between actors (i.e. those performing a task) and circumstances.

Errors may occur (see Figure 6.1):

- Due to the actor's
  - *Misperception*: information is incorrectly perceived, such that an incorrect intention is formed, and a wrong action performed. The intended action would have been correctly performed had the information been correctly perceived. For example, unintentional overdose may be caused by misreading the dose of an ampoule of adrenaline as 1:1000, rather than 1:100,000.
  - *Mistake*: information is correctly perceived, but an incorrect intention is formed, and a wrong action is performed. The intended action should have been correctly performed, given that the information was correctly perceived. For example, the ampoule of adrenaline was correctly read as 1:1000, but administered to a patient with malignant hypertension, resulting in a cerebrovascular accident.
  - *Slip*: information is correctly perceived, the correct intention is formed, but the wrong action is performed. The action is not what was intended. For example, the adrenaline is administered via an epidural catheter port, which is in close proximity to a central venous line port.
- Due to circumstance:
  - *Endogenous error*: that is error caused by the actor, relating to the circumstantial cause of aberrant mental processes that lead to misperceptions, mistakes, slips and distractions.

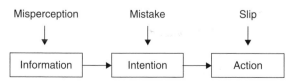

**Figure 6.1** The nature of errors caused by an actor.

    – *Exogenous error*: that is error caused by factors other than the actor, relating to, for example, product and systems design. If we accept that 'to err is human', then redesign of exogenous factors may be the best way of reducing error.
- Or due to a combination of actor and circumstance:
  - *errors of omission*, where an appropriate step of a process is left out;
  - *errors of insertion*, where an inappropriate step of a process is added;
  - *errors of repetition*, where an inappropriate step of a process (that is normally appropriate) is added;
  - *errors of substitution*, where an inappropriate step of a process is added, instead of an appropriate step.

In practice, medical errors can occur for a variety of pragmatic reasons:

1 Hospitals or general practices may offer services that they are not set up to provide competently. This may result from a number of factors, including underfunding, inadequate facilities or equipment, failures in management and difficulties recruiting or retaining appropriately trained staff.
2 They may result as a natural consequence of the process of medical training. A vital aspect of medical training is gaining the right sort of experience. This necessitates a practical learning process where students and junior staff members 'learn on the job'. Ideally this would require constant and adequate supervision. Nevertheless, the reality of the job is that this is not always the case and that, in any event, levels of experience and skill will vary from doctor to doctor, or nurse to nurse who occupy the same medical post or discharge the same duties.
3 Individuals may lack either sufficient confidence or competence to perform certain medical tasks reasonably. Individuals may be insufficiently or inadequately trained.
4 Difficult working conditions may give rise to an increased number of medical accidents. Shift work, fatigue, understaffing (relative or absolute) or excessive demand for healthcare have all been identified as contributory factors in medical accidents.
5 A 'brutalisation' of the medical profession may lead to a greater number of errors. The relatively modern notion of patients as 'consumers' of medical services and medical personnel as mere 'providers', has led to the suggestion that, to some extent, a depersonalised, production line mentality has come to influence the provision of medical services.

**6** Blame culture: If an undesirable outcome occurs, there is a modern tendency to try and identify the culpable. It has been noted that whilst medicine deals with shades of grey, the legal system sees only black and white. This may increasingly become the case as increasing numbers of professional standards and guidelines are introduced, which tend to assume that all patients will respond to a given treatment in a standard fashion, rather than in an individual way.

**7** Practitioners may adhere to outmoded forms of treatment, or may be forced to rely on outmoded forms because of budgetary constraints.

**8** Medical staff may fail to warn patients adequately (or at all) about the consequences of choosing certain medical procedures over others, or over no treatment at all. This may be due to time constraints, poor communication or medical uncertainty, but may also be a consequence of either a lack of training or doubt on the part of doctors in discharging or understanding their legal duties in this area.

**9** Inadequate communication between individuals or institutions may mean that similar, preventable errors continue to occur (e.g. recent legal cases involving the mistaken intrathecal injection of toxic anticancer drugs).

**10** Finally, there are often very different treatment regimes for the same or similar diseases. To some extent there is an element of experimentation with all patients concerning their treatment. For example, two different patients may present with the same disease but require slightly different forms of treatment because of their individual reaction to different drugs. The fundamentally experimental nature of medicine may result in errors occurring.

The ethical problem that arises essentially concerns whether people should be blamed, or held responsible, for their errors. The general concept behind the law of tort is that legal wrongs should be righted. Intuitively, this appeals to the idea that individuals should be held to account for the harm caused to others by their own carelessness. This adheres to the concept of moral blameworthiness, in that it is immoral to cause others harm through ones own carelessness: errors should be foreseen by the responsible actor before they occur, and actions voluntarily controlled to prevent their erroneous execution. Responsibility implies that errors occur because of flaws in character or behaviour. Nevertheless, if an adverse event occurs, there remains an injured patient, and it is commonly accepted in modern society that injured people, or the state, should not have to bear the burden of the faults of others, with society organised so that the deterrent effect of legal liability reduces risky and careless behaviour.

These general concepts, however, do provide for specific problems in medical negligence. It is arguable that legal 'fault' in negligence is not founded on moral blameworthiness. To be at fault in negligence one has to fail to meet the standard of the ordinary competent man. For example, a learner driver of a car on the road is expected to reach the standard of driving of the ordinary competent driver exercising the skill and competence of such a driver. For the purpose of the law of negligence, if the learner driver causes an accident it is not enough for the learner to say that they were doing their inexperienced best in a difficult situation. In such circumstances, it is difficult to attach moral blame when someone is judged by a hypothetical objective standard of expertise.

In medical negligence it may be hard to argue that the award of damages provides an effective deterrent to unreasonably risky activity. Firstly, civil litigation is such that damages may be awarded in a settlement of a claim to avoid legal cost or progress to court. So a determination or effective investigation into whether a particular course of conduct or activity was faulty and caused an injury may never occur. Thus lessons may not be learned or conduct altered. Moreover, it may be the case that there was no fault and that the procedure adopted was appropriate. It may be arguable that this reduces effective medical treatment to medical risk management. Secondly, in the UK health care is by and large paid for out of the public purse, and so litigation and compensation in the tort of negligence diverts resources from provision of medical care. It might be argued that these considerations mean that using the tort of negligence in medicine is unethical. Perhaps it would be better to invest in a system of complaint management or inquisition whereby medical errors can be independently investigated in a non-adversarial way where damages or compensation can be awarded, bad practice identified and medical staff effectively disciplined or retrained.

Ethical application of the tort of negligence to medical practice is therefore not as straightforward as initial instinctive reactions may suggest. Examination of the law concerning medical negligence reinforces these problems, as it illustrates the difficulty faced by injured patients in establishing a legal claim.

## LAW

Medical negligence occurs when there is a breach of a legal duty of care owed by a doctor (or health care professional) to a patient who they have undertaken to treat, that results in physical or mental damage or financial loss. Negligence actions are preferred by the courts in the UK when pursuing a cause of action, both because medical intent is not an issue (as the injury arises out of carelessness rather than deliberate action or recklessness), and because defendants are liable to pay financial damages to compensate for the damage caused by the negligence. Liability in negligence does not arise as a result of a pure accident.

Actions are usually brought under tort (i.e. a non-contractual civil wrong), because most UK doctors work for the NHS. By contrast private work is usually covered by contract law although concurrent liability in both contract and tort does arise in any event (and is not considered further here). Criminal negligence actions are still mercifully rare. However, there have been a number of successful prosecutions of doctors for gross negligence manslaughter recently.

According to the National Audit Office, 10,000 new claims of negligence against the NHS are made a year, with outstanding claims potentially liable for an estimated £2.6 billion. This represents a seven-fold increase compared to 5 years previously.

The rise in litigation does not necessarily represent doctors making more mistakes, although with increasingly invasive technology and treatment, the potential for injury is increased. Other factors operate: consumerism and media hysteria, together with a political desire for openness, tend to fuel a blame culture. Also, people are becoming more aware of their legal rights and appear more confident and ready to assert them. Publicity concerning large compensation awards seemingly encourages the aggrieved to seek legal redress. It should be noted, however, that only 25% of claims are successful. Furthermore, in 65% of claims settling for less than £50,000, legal and other expenses exceed the amount awarded. As previously alluded to, medicine operates in shades of grey. It is neither a true science as, in practice it can never guarantee forensic scientific certainty, nor is it a black and white subject like law. However, both the legal and medical professions are increasingly being asked to consider whether health care workers are either wholly right or wholly wrong.

A successful action in negligence requires the plaintiff (usually a patient) to establish the following:

- that a health care worker owed a duty of care to him/her;
- that the duty of care was breached;
- that the breach caused a foreseeable injury or damage to the claimant;
- that the health care worker could not avail themselves of a legal defence to the claim.

Duty and breach of duty may be reasonably easy to prove. However, most claims fail because the plaintiff fails to prove that the breach of duty caused their injury.

## Duty of care

Consider the following scenario: Mr X, a locum surgeon, performs a non-standard appendicectomy, after which the patient develops peritonitis and is placed on a high dependency unit because there are no beds available on the hospital's intensive care unit. The patient dies. In this setting, who, if anyone, may owe a duty of care to the patient? Two possibilities exist:

- *The doctor (Mr X)*: Doctors have a common law duty to their patient broadly when they undertake to help that patient. The existence of a duty may not be difficult to prove, although it may be more difficult to establish *when* a duty of care started (e.g. does the duty begin when Mr X actually sees the patient, or when the patient is referred to Mr X by his general practitioner (GP)?)
- *The hospital*: The liability of the hospital may be further subdivided into:
  - *Primary liability*: The hospital owes a duty both to provide a reasonable regime of care (a non-delegable duty that entails, for example providing proper facilities and equipment) and to ensure that reasonable care is taken (a non-delegable duty that entails, for example that agency staff and locums are adequately supervised and competent).
  - *Vicarious liability*: The hospital owes a duty of care to patients by ensuring that its doctors/employees are subjected to co-ordinated control and review of their work. NHS hospitals are subject to vicarious liability because they employ their staff (this may not be the case in private hospitals).

## Breach of duty of care

In order to succeed in negligence, a claimant must prove that it was more likely than not that the defendant did not exercise reasonable care in all the circumstances. In alleging a breach of duty, the claimant/patient must prove that the doctor failed to exercise the standard of care and skill expected of a reasonable professional holding themselves out to exercise such care and skill (e.g. an anaesthetist failing to monitor a patient according to a professional standard). This is easier to prove if there is an accepted or common practice, but less so if there is no standard practice (e.g. experimental treatments), or if the doctor practices non-standard therapies.

Originally, the standard of care expected of a doctor was assessed according to the *Bolam* test. In this case (*Bolam v Friern Hospital Management Committee* [1957] 2 All ER 118), after direction by the judge, a jury rejected Bolam's action that his fractured hip had been sustained through the negligent non-administration of a muscle relaxant during electro-convulsive therapy. The judge stated that:

> 'in the case of a medical man, negligence [breach of duty of care] means failure to act in accordance with the standards of reasonably competent medical men at the time'

This meant that normally a doctor could not be found negligent if (s)he was acting in accordance with a respectable body of medical opinion – if two schools of opinion existed, the doctor was not negligent if (s)he followed one of them (*Maynard v West Midlands RHA* [1985] 1 All ER 635 (HL)). Furthermore, according to *Sidaway* (*Sidaway v Bethlem Royal Hospital Governors* [1985] 1 All ER 643 (HL)), the 'standard of care is a matter of medical judgement'.

What is the effect of professional experience? In *Sidaway*, Lord Bridge declared that the standard of care is that of a specialist not just of a medical man – that is medical seniority imposes a higher standard of care. This was further considered in *Wilsher v Essex AHA* [1987] QB 730 (CA), where the standard of care expected of a junior doctor was dependent on the post which that junior occupied (i.e. a specialist registrar in cardiothoracic surgery owes a higher standard of care to a patient undergoing coronary artery bypass grafting than a specialist registrar in orthopaedics).

In an emergency, an inexperienced doctor may attempt procedures that a reasonable, inexperienced doctor may attempt (e.g. needle decompression of a tension pneumothorax, rather than thoracotomy!).

The advantages of the *Bolam* test are that it overcomes technical complexities, is valuable in questions of medical opinion and may be applied to all cases of diagnosis and treatment. However, by allowing doctors to determine what the standard of care is, the *Bolam* test is undoubtedly proscriptive in nature and overly deferential to the medical profession. In addition, the standard of care accepted may not necessarily equate to the best standard of care.

*Bolam* was reinterpreted by the House of Lords in *Bolitho v City and Hackney Health Authority* [1997] 4 All ER 771 (HL). In this case, the courts rejected two appeals by the mother of a deceased 2-year old that two doctors' failure both to attend and to intubate the boy for croup had resulted in the development of brain damage. Importantly, however,

*Bolitho* removed the determination of an acceptable standard of care from doctors, allowing courts the final say in the matter. In practice, peer assessment of clinical judgement is likely to continue to inform the standard of care. However, the *ratio* of *Bolitho* is that a court can decide, whether that body of medical opinion has informed the standard of care in a responsible, reasonable and respectable fashion.

As a result, practices which are based on habit, or are uninformed by medical progress, and which expose patients to excessive risk may become less defensible in negligence actions. This has been a driving force behind clinical standards agencies such as the National Institute of Clinical Excellence (NICE), whose evidence-based pronouncements are intended to guide doctors towards best clinical practice and away from irresponsible and unreasonable treatments. Guidelines are not law, but conduct that departs from the guidelines may increasingly be less amenable to legal defence.

But what about instances where there is no common practice? In *AB v Tameside and Glossop HA* [1997] 8 Med LR 91 (CA), the court determined that where there is no previous common practice, determination of the standard of care may be difficult (making it difficult for the claimant to prove a breach of duty), but the court should remain entitled to make enquiries anyway (applying *Bolitho* accordingly). The ultimate test in these circumstances is what the court determines as reasonable conduct in all of the circumstances of the case.

The question has arisen of whether lack of resources can find a defence to a negligence claim. For example, can the underfunding *per se* of an inadequately run intensive care unit provide a legal defence when a patient receives inadequate care, resulting in an injury. Kennedy and Grubb argue that the lack of resources cannot provide a defence for a claim in negligence. Once a hospital, for example, has opted to provide services and hold itself out to provide such services then they are required to exercise the care and skill of the ordinary competent hospital in providing those services, and a claim of lack of resources will not succeed. It is argued that issues of resources only relate to the initial decision whether or not to provide or withdraw services. Thus if an accident and emergency department is understaffed due to lack of staff or funding, it should withdraw from providing services to avoid liability in negligence. The provision of services is a matter of discretion for the government rather than in the tort of negligence (see Chapter 14).

## Causation and damages

It appears relatively straightforward for a claimant to prove that a doctor breached a duty of care. It is relatively more difficult to show that the breach of duty led to a specific injury. In general the law requires that the claimant prove that '*but for*' a doctors breach of duty of care injury and/or damage would not have occurred. The claimant, then, needs to show that the injury *could* have resulted from the breach of duty, and in fact *did* result from a breach of duty; it is generally insufficient to show that a breach of duty of care increased the risk of injury to the claimant (*Wilsher*). However, legal causation is a complex issue. Often there are multiple potential, cumulative, concurrent causes or alternative causes of an injury. Such causes can arise from a breach of duty of care or not. In such circumstances the law does not apply but for the test. It is enough, in the case of cumulative causes of an injury, that the claimant demonstrates that the breach of duty of care materially increased the risk of damage (*Bonnington Castings v Wardlaw* [1956] AC 613; *Wilsher*). In addition if there is a dispute concerning the medical evidence, that is an 'evidential gap', in these circumstances it may be enough for the claimant to demonstrate that the breach of duty materially contributed to the risk of their injury (*Fairchild* [2003] 1 AC 32, *McGhee* [1973] 1 WLR 1). However, the latter doctrine is applied sparingly (*Gregg v Scott* [2002] EWCA Civ 1471).

The law does not make the defendant liable for every outcome that occurred after the alleged breach – a surgeon who negligently per-forates small bowel during a laparoscopy that requires operative cor-rection by a second surgeon is not liable if the patient develops hospital-acquired pneumonia and multiple organ failure throughout a prolonged hospital stay. As Judge Kirby states in his analysis of negligent causation in the Australian case of *Chappel v Hart* [1998] 72 ALJR 1344 (HC of Aust)), 'causation is essentially a question of fact ... to be resolved as a matter of commonsense'. In practice, causation is a question of fact to be decided on the balance of probabilities.

If the claimant proves that a breach of duty was the sole cause, a sub-stantial cause or materially contributed to the injury, (s)he will succeed in claiming full damages. However, if (s)he fails to prove these, then the claim fails totally. The plaintiff must establish that 'but for' the negli-gence he would not have received any injury (and is awarded damages for all injuries), or that 'but for' the negligence (s)he would not have suffered an identifiable part or particular outcome of the injury (and is awarded damages for some of the injury), or that the negligence materi-ally contributed to the whole injury (e.g. failure to prescribe antibiotics for peritonitis that resulted from negligent bowel perforation) (*Tahir v Haringey HA* [1998] Lloyd's Rep Med 104 (CA)).

Pecuniary awards may be made for the harm occurring, for future financial burden and for the coverage of legal expenses. Section 100 of the Courts Act 2003 also allows for structured settlements, such that, rather than receiving a lump sum, the courts can order that the damages are paid as an periodical stipend (i.e. in instalments).

## Negligence in the provision of information

Doctors can be negligent when providing information to patients for the purpose of obtaining consent for treatment. Consent in the context of negligence differs to that required in the tort of battery. In battery, it is sufficient in broad terms to inform the patient of the nature and purpose of the procedure intended. To avoid a claim in negligence, however, may involve a significant discussion of the risks and consequences of treatment. Furthermore, a successful action in negligence requires that the patient prove that the breach of the duty to inform caused them damage. Namely, the patient must prove that the information given to them did not conform to an acceptable standard and that if the information had been given, the patient would not have consented to undergo the procedure.

Until recently, the courts have been reluctant to accept the arguments of claimants that they would not have undergone treatment had they been warned of the risks beforehand. This position may change in light of the recently decided case of *Chester v Afshar* [2002] EWCA Civ 724 (CA), in which the Court of Appeal held that:

> 'where, as a result of a doctor's failure to properly to advise a patient about the risk involved in a surgical procedure, the patient had an operation which she would not have otherwise have had at that time, and the risk materialised and caused her injury, the causal connection between the negligence and the damage was not broken merely because the patient had been unable to show that she would never, at any time in the future, have had an operation of that kind, carrying the same or similar risks'.

Such a decision is likely to influence moves toward increased information disclosure in future.

However, risks and consequences may occur unexpectedly, and have a very low prevalence. In addition, different patients attach different significance to different risks. The question arises as to whether doctors should adopt either a 'full disclosure' approach, informing patients of all the known risks and consequences, or a 'reasonable patient approach', which involves giving information to which a reasonable patient in the patient's condition would be likely to attach significance (e.g. the risk of vocal cord damage when at intubation for opera singers). In *Sidaway*, the majority applied *Bolam* to information disclosure (i.e. the standard of disclosure should be in accordance with the acceptable medical standards of the time), although Lord Scarman appeared to favour the reasonable patient standard. The effect of *Bolitho* is that non-disclosure of information would not be deemed negligent if the reason for non-disclosure was reasonable, responsible and rational. *Pearce* (*Pearce v United Bristol Healthcare Trust* [1998] 48 BMLR 118 (CA)), a case which considered *Sidaway* in the light of *Bolitho*, determined that a doctor would be negligent if disclosure was so obviously necessary to an informed choice, that no reasonable medical man would fail to disclose the information.

It should also be noted that there may be an additional duty to disclose information beyond the risks and consequences of a procedure (e.g. the risks and consequences of *not* operating, the possibility of other therapies, information about the surgeon (e.g. human immunodeficiency virus (HIV) status), hospital mortality rates, etc. – all of which may materially contribute to a patient's final decision to give consent), although UK case law is deficient in this area at present.

Finally, doctors have a duty to answer questions from patients, and truthfully (*Sidaway*). Similarly, doctors have a duty to inform patients if a treatment has failed or has gone wrong (*AB v Tameside and Glossop*).

## Medical error and The Clinical Negligence Scheme for Trusts

Errors are a predictable function of work, and a certain amount of error is routine in any area of work. This is particularly the case with work that involves human interaction (such as the practice of medicine), when the basis of action is often human opinion. Traditionally, investigations into medical errors (which have the potential to seriously harm patients) have sought to focus blame on individuals or institutions – indeed, this is the method by which the law operates in deciding medical negligence claims. The problem with this approach is that the legal apportioning of blame is equated by the public with guilt and incompetence on the part of the doctor. This ignores both the psychology of human nature, and the fact that doctors (by and large) never set out with the intention of harming their patients. The production of legal 'scapegoats', some authors have argued, does not address the underlying problem of faulty systems. For example, over the last decade there have been a number of incidents of inexperienced doctors injecting anticancer drugs into the intrathecal space of patients with cancer, with disastrous and often fatal consequences. In these cases, blame has been apportioned both to the institutions and to the doctors involved; indeed, in legal terms, the doctors may have been negligent for failing to meet an acceptable standard of care, the institutions primarily or vicariously liable in negligence for failing to provide a reasonable regime of care, or for failing to inform the actions of their doctors. However, the mistakes keep on occurring – so is the mistake a fault of the doctor, or is it intrinsic to the process of delivering intrathecal chemotherapy?

Two other points should be made. Firstly, some authors have highlighted that a blame culture is counterproductive – it encourages defensive medicine (i.e. medical practice which aims to minimise legal liability rather than provide better, but riskier, treatment for patients), to the detriment of patients, as well as acting as a disincentive to medical personnel to report errors, to the detriment of current *and future* patients. The development of 'no fault compensation' has arisen in recognition of this position.

Secondly, it must be noted that a paradigm shift away from 'blame' to 'no fault' should not seek to provide a shield behind which seriously negligent medical practices can hide. Medicine is a responsible profession, held in trust by the public, and should be seen to distinguish between negligence worthy of reprimand, and straightforward error, worthy of repair.

The above approaches are to some extent reflected by the Clinical Negligence Scheme for Trusts (CNST). Alarmed at the rising cost of negligence litigation, the CNST was established in 1994, and deals with claims arising after the 1 April 1995. The NHS Litigation Authority (NHSLA – a special health authority) administers the scheme, which is voluntary and open to all NHS trusts. Basically, NHSLA assessors predict the total payout costs of litigation per year and divide this by the number of trusts in the scheme, to produce a figure payable per Trust per year. The final amount payable is then adjusted according to size of hospital, activities, budget, etc. The innovative component of this scheme is that trusts can qualify for a reduction of payments of up to 30% if they meet certain risk management standards, which include for example, critical incident reporting, and the development and implementation of policies and procedures. It is hoped that by applying local financial incentives that clinical risk management will improve on a national basis, although this remains to be seen.

## FURTHER READING

### Books

Green M and McConnochie K. *Clinical Negligence and Complaints: a Clinician's Guide.*
    RSM press, London, 2002
Institute of Medicine. *To Err is Human: Building a Safety Health System.* National
    Academy Press, Washington, 1999

Mason JK and Smith MRA (Eds). Medical Negligence. In: *Law and Medical Ethics*, 5th
    edition. Chapter 9, pp. 215–240
Kennedy I and Grubb A (Eds). Medical Negligence. In: *Medical Law*, 3rd edition. Chapter
    4, pp. 271–574
Merry A and Smith MRA. *Errors, Medicine and the Law*. Cambridge University Press,
    Cambridge, 2001


## Journals

Barach P and Small SD. Reporting and preventing medical mishaps: lessons from
    non-medical near miss reporting systems. *Br Med J* 2000; **320**: 759–763
Brazier M and Miola J. Bye-bye Bolam: a medical litigation revolution? *Med Law Rev*
    2000; **8**: 85–111
Capstick B. The future of clinical negligence litigation? *Br Med J* 2004; **328**: 457–459
Fenn P, Diacon S, Gray A, Hodges R and Rickman N. Current cost of medical negligence
    in NHS hospitals: analysis of claims database. *Br Med J* 2000; **320**: 1567–1571
Leape LL. Error in medicine. *J Am Med Assoc* 1994; **272**: 1151–1157
Mayberry MK. Effects of the civil procedure rules on clinical negligence claims. *Postgrad
    Med J* 2003; **79**: 74–77
Samanta A, Samanta J and Gunn M. Legal considerations of clinical guidelines: will NICE
    make a difference? *J Roy Soc Med* 2003; **96**: 133–138


## Internet

British Medical Association. Duty of candour?
    http://www.bma.org.uk/ap.nsf/Content/Duty+of+candour%3F
Department of Health. Clinical Negligence. What are the issues and options for reform?
    http://www.doh.gov.uk/clinicalnegligencereform/
Department of Health. An organisation with a memory. Report of an expert group on
    learning from adverse events in the NHS. The Stationery Office, London, 2000.
    http://www.publications.doh.gov.uk/orgmemreport/
General Medical Council. Good Medical Practice, 2001.
    http://www.gmc-uk.org/standards/good.htm
Healthcare Commission. http://www.healthcarecommission.org.uk/Homepage/fs/en
National Audit Office. Handling Clinical Negligence Claims in England. May, 2001.
    http://www.nao.gov.uk/publications/nao_reports/00-01/0001403.pdf
National Clinical Assessment Authority. http://www.ncaa.nhs.uk/
National Patient Safety Agency. http://www.npsa.nhs.uk/
NHS Litigation Authority. Clinical Negligence Scheme for Trusts. Clinical risk
    management standards. http://www.willis.com/NHSLA/attachments/
    General%20Manual%20June%202002.pdf

# 7
# Confidentiality, and access to medical records

*'What I may see or hear in the course of the treatment or even outside of the treatment in regard to the life of men, which on no account one must spread abroad, I will keep to myself, holding such things shameful to be spoken about'*
– the Hippocratic Oath

*'Patients have a right to expect that doctors will not disclose any personal information which they learn during the course of their professional duties, unless they give permission'*
– General Medical Council (GMC), 'Duties of a Doctor'

Modern medical practice is founded on the concept of respecting patient autonomy, which in part includes respecting the right of an individual to determine what personal information may or may not be divulged to a third party. Unwarranted disclosure of a patient's medical treatment, advice or medical records is regarded as breach of their personal integrity. In essence, confidentiality protects the patient's informational autonomy.

The concepts of confidentiality and privacy are inter-related, but they are not identical. Privacy is generally viewed as an individual right, whereas confidentiality is considered an interest but not necessarily an individual right.

The major ethical theories accommodate the notion of confidentiality. Deontology envisages confidentiality as a moral duty, but accepts that breaching confidentiality may be ethically acceptable if there is a more pressing duty to disclose information. Utilitarianism supports confidentiality if it promotes the best consequences, but obviously allows for breaches of confidentiality if the greater good is best served by disclosure. The maintenance of confidentiality may also be seen as a virtue in its own right.

Public or community interests may be best served by confidentiality, or the forming of confidential relationships (e.g. doctor–patient, solicitor–client, priest–parishioner). The interest here is that the community realises the importance of keeping certain types of information confidential, rather than having the information disclosed. Naturally, there are circumstances in which the community interest in confidentiality competes with a similar community interest in disclosure.

In terms of medical confidentiality, community interests are preserved by people being able to seek medical help and treatment without details of their medical treatment becoming widely disseminated. It is argued that people would be reluctant to seek such help. Confidentiality enhances trust and co-operation between the patient and the medical practitioner. However, this interest is not absolute and under certain specified circumstances, the medical practitioner owes a greater duty to the general community than the individual they are treating. In these circumstances the medical practitioner may be obliged or has the discretion to breach any obligation of confidence they may owe a patient. The ethical dilemma that this creates for a medical practitioner is where and when can they legally and ethically breach this duty of confidence.

## LAW

Confidentiality is the key cornerstone of a trusting doctor–patient relationship. This concern is reflected by professional ethical guidelines, including the Hippocratic Oath and the GMC's *Duties of a Doctor*, and by the seriousness that the law attaches to the legal duty of confidentiality. The implementation of both the Human Rights Act, 1998 (HRA) (Article 8 of which concerns the right to respect for private and family life) and the Data Protection Act, 1998 (DPA) reinforces the importance of the duty of confidentiality in medical practice.

The DPA prescribes the statutory relationship between 'data subjects' (namely patients), 'data controllers' (including hospitals) and 'data processors' (including doctors) and regulates access to personal information, penalties for breaches of confidentiality and circumstances in which confidentiality may be breached. A data subject's physical or mental health condition is classified as 'sensitive personal data'. Eight data protection principles are described in schedules to the DPA (see Figure 7.1).

The common law of confidentiality has effectively been incorporated into the first data protection principle through the concept of data being 'processed ... lawfully'. In order to understand the statutory legal protection of personal data, therefore, one must understand the common law of confidentiality. Moreover, the common law of confidentiality remains a powerful tool affording protection to confidential medical information that is not contained in a 'health record' (as defined by Section 68 of the DPA, 1998).

1   Personal data shall be processed fairly and lawfully and, in particular, shall not be processed unless
    (a) at least one of the conditions in Schedule 2 is met;
    (b) in the case of sensitive personal data, at least one of the condition in Schedule 3 is also met.

2   Personal data shall be obtained only for one or more specified and lawful purposes, and shall not be further processed in any manner incompatible with that purpose or those purposes.

3   Personal data shall be adequate, relevant and not excessive in relation to the purpose or purposes for which they are processed.

4   Personal data shall be accurate and, where necessary, kept up to date.

5   Personal data processed for any purpose or purposes shall not be kept for longer than is necessary for that purpose or those purposes.

6   Personal data shall be processed in accordance with the rights of data subjects under this act.

7   Appropriate technical and organisational measures shall be taken against unauthorised or unlawful processing of personal data and against accidental loss or destruction of or damage to, personal data.

8   Personal data shall not be transferred to a country or territory outside the European Economic Area unless that country or territory ensures an adequate level of protection for the rights and freedoms of data subjects in relation to the processing of personal data.

**Figure 7.1**  The eight data protection principles of the DPA.

## Common law: a legal duty of confidentiality

When does a duty of confidence arise in common law? This duty was formulated by Lord Goff in the 'Spycatcher' case (*A-G v Guardian Newspapers (No 2)* [1990] 1 AC 109), who stated that a 'duty of confidence arises when confidential information comes to the knowledge of a person … that the information is confidential … such that (the confidant) should be precluded from disclosing the information to others'.

The duty of medical confidence was similarly confirmed in the case of *W v Egdell* [1990] 1 All ER 835 (CA), when Bingham LJ referred to GMC's advice to doctors pursuant to Section 35 of the Medical Act, 1983, as being the general rule of law:

'It is a doctor's duty … strictly to observe the rule of professional secrecy by refraining from disclosing voluntarily to any third party, information about a patient which he has learnt directly or indirectly in his professional capacity as a registered medical practitioner'.

Furthermore, the law of confidence extends such that doctors should not disclose information learnt either directly, or from other sources in his persona as the patient's doctor (e.g. second-hand medical information relayed by a patient's relative). Therefore, doctors must not breach their duty of confidentiality in order to disclose information, for example, to employers, insurance companies or third parties. This duty of confidentiality extends to children, the dead and incompetent adults (although it has been suggested that no duty exists if the person has always been incompetent because a confidential relationship could never have developed).

However, in England and Wales the law of confidentiality has traditionally concerned itself more with protecting the public interest, rather than with individual rights. The balance has been less in favour of protecting the public interest in maintaining individual confidences, compared to the greater weight accorded to the public interest disclosure of purportedly confidential information. Since the law of confidentiality is linked to concepts of the public interest, the duty of medical confidentiality is not absolute. There are certain conditions under which confidentiality may be waived or breached, including several statutory instances requiring disclosure of confidential information. It is always the case at common law that a duty of confidentiality can be lawfully breached or waived with the consent of a competent patient.

## When may confidentiality be breached?

In general, the duty of confidentiality can be breached:

- *With the patient's consent*: This takes into account the common law of consent, such that the patient must be competent to give informed consent, voluntarily. Consent to disclosure may be expressed (e.g. written consent for disclosure of medical records for insurance purposes) or implied (e.g. by not objecting when a doctor tells a patient that he needs to discuss their case with a medical colleague). However, there may be natural limitations on the extent of disclosure even with lawful consent. For example, a patient may consent to disclosure of confidential information, but this may only extend to other medical staff necessarily involved in their treatment, rather than additionally to the media. The law concerning circumstances of consent to breach or waiver of confidentiality on the part of children and incompetent adults remains underdeveloped. It appears that for children, they can be presumed to enter into a confidential relationship when they have the requisite capacity *per Gillick*; alternatively that confidentiality may operate and be limited by proxies acting in the child's best interest. It may be the case with incompetent adults that the law presumes they are owed a duty of confidence and that this confidentiality may be breached and limited by the doctrine of necessity with regard to their medical best interests.

- *When it is in the public interest*: When the public interest in disclosure of information imparted in confidence outweighs the public interest in non-disclosure (*X v Y* [1988] 2 All ER 648 (QBD)). This may happen in one of the four following circumstances:

  - When there is a danger to the health or safety of others, but only if this a real, rather than a fanciful, risk of harm. This may include the knowing transmission of serious communicable diseases, including human immunodeficiency virus (HIV).
  - In order to detect or prevent *serious* crime.
  - For the purposes of teaching, research or auditing (although the GMC suggests that data should be anonymised and disclosed after obtaining consent, wherever possible).
  - For National Health Service (NHS) administration or management purposes (although the GMC suggests that financial and administrative data should be held separately to clinical data).

- According to the following:
  - Statutory provision, including:
    (a) Section 11 Public Health (Control of Diseases) Act, 1984 – notifiable diseases. Doctors have a duty to inform the Local Authority's Medical Officer for Environmental Health if a patient has a 'notifiable disease' (see Figure 7.2). The

| Notifiable diseases, according to<br>Public Health (Control of Disease) Act, 1984 | |
| --- | --- |
| Acute encephalitis | Ophthalmia neonatorum |
| Acute meningitis | Paratyphoid A or B |
| Anthrax | Plague |
| Cholera | Polio |
| Continued fever | Puerperal fever |
| Diphtheria | Rabies |
| Dysentery | Relapsing fever |
| Erysipelas | Scarlet fever |
| Food poisoning | Smallpox |
| Lassa fever | Tetanus |
| Leprosy | Tuberculosis (TB) |
| Leptospiral jaundice | Typhoid fever |
| Malaria | Typhus fever |
| Marburg virus disease | Viral hepatitis |
| Measles | Viral haemorrhagic fever |
| Membranous croup | Whooping cough |
| Meningococcal infection | Yellow fever |

**Figure 7.2** Notifiable diseases.

information that should be provided includes: name, age, sex, address, disease (confirmed or suspected), its date of onset, hospital admission date and doctors opinion as to whether the disease was acquired in hospital;

(b) Regulation 5 Abortion Regulations, 1991;

(c) Regulation 2 NHS (Venereal Diseases) Regulations, 1974;

(d) Misuse of Drugs Act, 1973 – drug addiction;

(e) Medical Act, 1983 (allows disclosure of information to the GMC in respect of its powers to investigate complaints against doctors);

(f) Prevention of Terrorism Act, 1989;

(g) Audit Commission Act, 1998 (allowing the Audit Commission to carry out its work);

(h) Road Traffic Act, 1988 – name and address (only) of driver allegedly guilty of offence under this act.

- A court order or search warrant signed by a court judge.

In all cases, disclosure should only be made to the relevant person or authority. It is rare for legal authority to allow unlimited disclosure, although if confidential information is in the public domain, the law will be slow to intervene to restrain its further disclosure and dissemination.

Unauthorised and unlawful breaches of confidentiality are normally prevented by the data subject seeking an injunction against the data controller. An injunction is a court order designed to prevent the subject of the order from doing certain things. Breaching the terms of a valid injunction can lead to a claim of contempt of court, which could lead to the imprisonment of the contemnor.

There are other remedies available to patients after an unauthorised breach of confidentiality. In law, breach of a personal confidence is analogous to that of breach of a commercial confidence. Damages may be sought (but not necessarily awarded) if the breach of confidence caused the data subject harm, despite the reluctance of Judge Scott in *W v Egdell* to recognise shock and distress as harmful consequences of a breach of confidentiality.

## The Data Protection Act, 1998

The implementation of the DPA and the HRA has effected a change in the legal ownership of personal data. As a result, almost all information that comprises personal data is legally owned by the data subject. The DPA not only impacts on medical treatment and record keeping, but

---

**SCHEDULE 2**
**Conditions relevant for purposes of the first principle:**
**processing of any personal data**

1   The data subject has given his consent to the processing.

2   The processing is necessary:
(a) for the performance of a contract to which the data subject is a party,
(b) for the taking of steps at the request of the data subject with a view to entering into a contract.

3   The processing is necessary for compliance with any legal obligation to which the data controller is subject, other than an obligation imposed by contract.

4   The processing is necessary in order to protect the vital interests of the data subject.

5   The processing is necessary:
(a) for the administration of justice,
(b) for the exercise of any functions conferred on any person by or under any enactment,
(c) for the exercise of any functions of the Crown, a Minister of the Crown or a government department,
(d) for the exercise of any other functions of a public nature exercised in the public interest by any person.

6   (1) The processing is necessary for the purposes of legitimate interests pursued by the data controller or by the third party or parties to whom the data are disclosed, except where the processing is unwarranted in any particular case by reason of prejudice to the rights and freedoms or legitimate interests of the data subject.
(2) The Secretary of State may by order specify particular circumstances in which this condition is, or is not, to be taken to be satisfied.

---

**Figure 7.3** Schedule 2 provisions of the DPA.

also on research and cancer registries. In the DPA, 'information relating to an individual's physical or mental condition' constitutes 'sensitive personal data', where the most stringent conditions of the DPA apply. Such data must be processed 'fairly and lawfully'. There is no exhaustive definition of what 'fairly' or 'lawfully' means in the DPA, but it encompasses the notion of confidentiality. The act states that in order to process sensitive information fairly and lawfully, at least one condition from Schedule 2 and one from Schedule 3 to the act must be fulfilled (see Figures 7.3 and 7.4).

The conditions in Schedule 2 include patient consent, the necessity of processing for the exercise of any functions of the Crown, a Minister of the Crown or a government department, and the necessity of processing for the exercise of any functions of a public nature exercised in the public interest by any person.

*Inter alia*, Schedule 3 requires that 'processing is necessary for medical purposes'. Here 'medical purposes' are broadly defined to include

---

**SCHEDULE 3**
**Conditions relevant for purposes of the first principle:**
**processing of sensitive personal data**

1   The data subject has given his explicit consent to the processing of the
    personal data.

8       (1) The processing is necessary for medical purposes and is undertaken by:
            (a) a health professional,
            (b) a person who in the circumstances owes a duty of confidentiality which
                is equivalent to that which would arise if that person were a health
                professional.
        (2) In this paragraph 'medical purposes' includes the purposes of preventative
            medicine, medical diagnosis, medical research, the provision of care and
            treatment and the management of health care services.

---

**Figure 7.4**  Relevant sections of Schedule 3 of the DPA.

purposes of preventative medicine, medical diagnosis, research, the
provision of care and treatment and the management of medical health
care services.

## Human rights, privacy and confidentiality

Personal information that is held in confidence is protected by Article
8(1) of the European Convention of Human Rights (ECHR), as incorporated by HRA. The right protected here is an individual's 'right of respect
for his private and family life'. Any disclosure of confidential information
must be justified according to Article 8(2) of the ECHR as being:

(a)   in accordance with the law;
(b)   necessary in a democratic society, that is, proportionate;
(c)   for a stated purpose: in the interests of public safety, for economic
      well-being of the country, for the prevention of crime and
      disorder, for the protection of health and morals or for the
      protection of rights and freedoms of others.

Article 8 of the ECHR codifies the nature of a public interest that
might justify a breach of confidentiality by a public body (such as the
NHS). Section 6 of the HRA requires the NHS to act compatibly with
the ECHR. In *A Health Authority v X* [2001] Lloyd's Rep Med 349,
Mr Justice Munby held that the disclosure of a patient's records to a
health authority for disciplinary and regulatory purposes was justified
under Article 8, provided that the records remained confidential and that
express conditions were in place to prevent their disclosure. The court

remains the ultimate arbiter of whether the public interest is best served by disclosure or confidentiality.

## Health and Social Care Act 2001

Section 60 of the Health and Social Care Act, 2001 was introduced to resolve problems caused by the DPA, concerning issues of confidentiality. The act enables the Secretary of State to make certain regulations (subject to a series of safeguards) that bypass the general rule requiring patient's consent for the disclosure of information. Regulations include the authority to disclose confidential information 'where essential services cannot, having regard to present NHS systems and available technology, operate on (an informed consent) basis' (Explanatory notes to the act, Paragraph 291), and power to compel NHS bodies to disclose confidential patient information to certain persons. These regulations, for example, could be used to make cancer a notifiable disease, requiring communication of new patients to registries.

The Health Service (Control of Patient Information) Regulations 2002 have already been passed under the act, which authorise the procurement of otherwise confidential patient information from patients referred for the 'diagnosis or treatment of neoplasia' (cancer research provisions) and any patient where processing is 'with a view to diagnosing communicable diseases and other risks to public health'. Where the Secretary of State considers it necessary to process information for public health purposes, they may serve a notice on a health care worker with a penalty of up to £5000 if they fail to comply.

## Access to medical records

The maintenance of contemporaneous, accurate and clear medical records is an essential part of perioperative medicine. Particularly at a time of ever-increasing patient throughput, medical records act as a valuable *aide-memoire* for the clinician. More importantly, they are a vital form of communication between clinicians involved in the continued care of a patient. As such, there is a degree of moral necessity attached to their maintenance, as part of providing the very best in medical care. Moreover, there would appear to be a legal obligation owed by perioperative physicians to their patients to maintain good medical records.

Normally, medical records (which may be written or stored electronically) are a matter between the patient and his/her doctor or doctors (or allied health professionals) concerned with the direct provision of care to that patient. However, two situations may arise that modify the normal relationship between the 'medical data holder' (i.e. the doctor) and the 'medical data subject' (i.e. the patient):

- the patient may wish to see his/her medical records;
- a third party may wish to see the medical records.

Prior to the passage of the Administration of Justice Act, 1970 (Sections 32–35), medical records were not accessible by either patient or third party in advance of a court trial. The 1970 Act empowered the court to order the disclosure of any medical records that were relevant to the evidence of a case. Once the conceptual shift had been established allowing their compulsory disclosure, medical records became increasingly accessible.

Further statutory provisions concerning disclosure soon followed. Section 35 of the Supreme Court Act, 1981 empowered the court to refuse to order disclosure that might be injurious to the public interest. The Data Protection Act, 1984 (repealed by DPA, 1998) was introduced in order to comply with European legislation, and enabled patients to view information held about them on computer. The Access to Medical Reports Act, 1988 established a right of access for individuals to reports relating to themselves provided by medical practitioners for employment or insurance purposes.

Finally, the Access to Health Records Act, 1990 extended the right of individuals to medical records kept manually (and made after 1 November, 1991), and provided for the correction of inaccurate health records. This act gave patients the general right to see any of their medical records, obtain copies of these records and have their records explained to them, although the record-holder (i.e. the doctor) retained a discretionary right to withhold information that (s)he believed might be seriously detrimental to the physical or mental health of the patient. In addition, doctors had to ensure that the confidentiality of other (non-medical) persons was maintained – records relating, for example, to spouses or other relatives could be deleted without informing the patient (although the patient was permitted to enquire whether these notes had been deleted). The record-holder had to produce the notes (or copies) for the patient within 21 days, for which the record-holder could charge a fee for the costs of production.

Concerns over the secure use of patient data held by the NHS led to a review commissioned by the Chief Medical Officer, which resulted in the Caldicott Report 1997. Six key principles were identified (Figure 7.5), and 16 selected recommendations made (Figure 7.6), aimed at providing a clear framework for the storage and use of patient data. Recommendation 3 called for the nomination of 'a senior person' in each health

**Principle 1.** *Justify the purpose(s).*
Every proposed use or transfer of patient identifiable information within or from an organisation should be clearly defined and scrutinised with continuing uses regularly reviewed, by an appropriate guardian.

**Principle 2.** *Don't use patient identifiable information unless it is absolutely necessary.*
Patient identifiable information items should not be included unless it is essential for the specified purpose(s) of that flow. The need for patients to be identified should be considered at each stage of satisfying the purpose(s).

**Principle 3.** *Use the minimum necessary patient – identifiable information.*
Where use of patient identifiable information is considered to be essential, the inclusion of each individual item of information should be considered and justified so that the minimum amount of identifiable information is transferred or accessible as is necessary for a given function to be carried out.

**Principle 4.** *Access to patient identifiable information should be on a strict need to know basis.*
Only those individuals who need access to patient identifiable information should have access to it and they should only have access to the information items that they need to see. This may mean introducing access controls or splitting information flows where one information flow is used for several purposes.

**Principle 5.** *Everyone with access to patient identifiable information should be aware of their responsibilities.*
Action should be taken to ensure that those handling patient identifiable information – both clinical and non-clinical staff – are made fully aware of their responsibilities and obligations to respect patient confidentiality.

**Principle 6.** *Understand and comply with the law.*
Every use of patient identifiable information must be lawful. Someone in each organization, handling patient information should be responsible for ensuring that the organisation complies with legal requirements.

**Figure 7.5** The six key principles of data handling within the NHS (Caldicott Report, 1997).

organisation to act as a guardian (a 'Caldicott guardian') responsible for safeguarding the confidentiality of patient information.

Although they are not law, the principles provide a sound basis for good practice when handling data in perioperative settings as they do for other areas of medicine.

In order to give effect to the European Directive on Personal Data 1995 (OJ L281), both the Access to Health Records Act, 1990 and the Access to Medical Reports Act, 1988 have been effectively repealed by the DPA (*vide supra*), which governs access to *all* medical records, whether written or electronic, and whenever they were created.

The sole remaining basis for access to medical records under the Access to Health Records Act, 1990 relates to the ability of relatives or concerned individuals to access the records of a dead patient, when that

1   Every dataflow, current or proposed, should be tested against basic principles of good practice. Continuing flows should be re-tested regularly.

2   A programme of work should be established to reinforce awareness of confidentiality and information security requirements amongst all staff within the NHS.

3   A senior person, preferably a health professional, should be nominated in each health organisation to act as a guardian, responsible for safeguarding the confidentiality of patient information.

5   Protocols should be developed to protect the exchange of patient-identifiable information between NHS and non-NHS bodies.

6   The identity of those responsible for monitoring the sharing and transfer of information within agreed local protocols should be clearly communicated.

9   Strict protocols should define who is authorised to gain access to patient identity where the NHS number or other coded identifier is used.

10   Where particularly sensitive information is transferred, privacy enhancing technologies (e.g. encrypting identifiers or 'patient identifying information') must be explored.

11   Those involved in developing health information systems should ensure that best practice principles are incorporated during the design stage.

**Figure 7.6** Selected recommendations of the Caldicott Report, 1997.

access is relevant to legal action arising out of the patient's death (Sections 3(1)f and 3(2)).

Section 7 of the DPA governs the rights of data subjects and others to access medical records (Figure 7.7). In essence:

- patients should be informed:
  - if the data controller intends to disclose confidential medical information;
  - to whom the data is being disclosed, and why;
  - in an intelligible fashion if they enquire about information held as a personal medical record.

- data controllers are not obliged to disclose the contents of medical records (e.g. for insurance purposes):
  - unless they receive the request in writing, with verification of the patient's consent to disclosure;
  - usually unless a suitable fee is paid;
  - if they are not confident that third party anonymity will be maintained (without the consent of that third party);

- the courts may order the data controller to disclose medical records if they are not satisfied with the data controllers' reasons for non-disclosure;

---

**Data Protection Act, 1998**
**Rights of data subject and others**

7  (1)  Subject to the following provisions of this section ..., an individual is entitled
   (a)  to be informed by any data controller whether personal data of which that individual is the data subject are being processed by or on behalf of that data controller;
   (b)  if that is the case, to be given by the data controller a description of;
       (i)  the personal data of which that individual is the data subject,
       (ii)  the purposes for which they are being or are to be processed,
       (iii)  the recipients or classes of recipients to whom they are or may be disclosed.
   (c)  to have communicated to him in an intelligible form;
       (i)  the information constituting any personal data of which that individual is the data subject,
       (ii)  any information available to the data controller as to the source of those data,

   (2)  A data controller is not obliged to supply any information under subsection (1) unless he has received;
   (a)  a request in writing,
   (b)  except in prescribed cases, such fee (not exceeding the prescribed maximum) as he may require.

   (3)  A data controller is not obliged to comply with a request under this section unless he is supplied with such information as he may reasonably require in order to satisfy himself as to the identity of the person making the request and to locate the information which that person seeks;

   (4)  Where a data controller cannot comply with the request without disclosing information relating to another individual who can be identified from that information, he is not obliged to comply with the request unless;
   (a)  the other individual has consented to the disclosure of the information to the person making the request,
   (b)  it is reasonable in all the circumstances to comply with the request without the consent of the other individual.

   (9)  If a court is satisfied on the application of any person who has made a request under the foregoing provisions of this section that the data controller in question has failed to comply with the request in contravention of those provisions, the court may order him to comply with the request.

**Figure 7.7** The rights of data subjects (patients) and others, regarding data access, according to the DPA.

- the Secretary of State for Health (to whom doctors can apply for an exemption) retains a right to exempt patients from accessing their records if disclosure '*would be likely* to cause *serious* harm to the physical or mental health or condition of the data subject *or any persons*' – note the italics (Article 5(1) of the Data Protection (Subject Access Modification)(Health) Order 2000 (SI 2000, No 413)).

However, that data subjects are allowed access to their personal data does not imply that they are allowed access to *all* personal medical data. In addition to the above, other restrictions include:

- data that is held or processed for research, statistical or historical purposes, provided the data is anonymous, not intended to influence decisions about the patient and that data processing is not likely to cause substantial damage or distress to the patient (Section 33). Concerns have recently been expressed that the DPA is unnecessarily obstructive to the course of research, particularly epidemiological research because of the necessity of protecting individual confidentiality.
- when a regulatory role is involved – that is the GMC and the Commission for Healthcare Audit and Inspection (CHAI) may process medical records, for example, in order to protect the public from incompetent or dishonest doctors or practices (Section 31).

According to the DPA, three remedies are available to data subjects with regards to the improper use of their personal data by a data controller:

- the data subject can ask the data controller to cease data processing, or apply to the court to order this (Section 10);
- the data subject may seek compensation for damage caused as a result of the data controllers' obligations (Section 13);
- the court may ask the data controller to rectify, block, erase or destroy inaccurate data or opinion about the data subject (Section 14).

The DPA is less forthcoming about applications for medical data disclosure made on behalf of children or incompetent adults (e.g. by the relatives of an unconscious patient on the intensive care unit). Unlike the Access to Health Records Act, 1990, there is no specific section that deals with this scenario. Kennedy and Grubb ('*Medical Law*', 3rd ed., p. 1028) suggest that the provisions described under Section 7 of the DPA are either strict, such that only competent child or adult patients may ever apply for access to their medical records (which therefore precludes disclosure to relatives if the child or adult is incompetent) or that medical data may be requested by a third party (relative), but only released to the data subject – which is pointless if the data subject is unconscious. It is not enough for disclosure to be in the patient's best interests. Kennedy and Grubb point out that disclosure to third parties could be justified, if:

- the third parties were formally identified as potential recipients;
- the doctor complied with the data protection principles, such that disclosure was 'fair' and 'necessary to protect the vital interests of

the data subject' (i.e. to prevent death or critical deterioration of the patient) or 'necessary for medical purposes' (i.e. to further critical treatment of the patient).

Kennedy and Grubb suggest that necessity may be a weaker defence when disclosing sensitive personal data about adult incompetents, because ordinarily relatives have no legal power to make medical treatment decisions about them (this situation may change in light of the proposed Mental Incapacity Bill – see Chapter 5), although they point out that 'consultation with relatives about the medical treatment of an incompetent adult is good/best practice. Disclosure is, consequently, an adjunct to the treatment of the patient.'

There remains an obligation to keep medical data confidential after the death of a patient, although disclosure may be warranted:

- with the patient's premortem consent;
- where a parent seeks information about the circumstances of their child's death;
- if confidential information about the patient or identifiable third parties is anonymised;
- if disclosure is necessary to protect the deceased's vital interests (e.g. pertains to ongoing financial considerations);
- in order to complete a death certificate;
- if disclosure is ordered by the courts or is required by a coroner in order to assist with an inquest or fatal accident inquiry or is required for official audit or education purposes (e.g. National Confidential Enquiries, such as National Confidential Enquiry into Perioperative Death, NCEPOD).

To what extent does the patient control the information contained in their medical records, such that the information cannot be disclosed without the patient's consent? This has been largely covered in the first part of this chapter, in the analysis of the provisions of the DPA. However, it is worth reiterating some of those provisions with relevance to the patient's control of their medical records:

- all health records, whether written or electronic, are covered;
- 'information relating to an individual's physical or mental condition' constitutes 'sensitive personal data';
- sensitive personal data must be processed 'fairly and lawfully';
- in order to process (i.e. disclose) sensitive information fairly and lawfully at least one condition from Schedule 2 and one from Schedule 3 to the act must be fulfilled (Figures 7.3 and 7.4);

- Schedule 2 conditions include patient consent and the necessity of disclosure for legal reasons;
- Schedule 3 requires that 'processing is necessary for medical purposes', including purposes of medical diagnosis, research, the provision of care and treatment and the management of medical health care services.

The GMC have incorporated both the findings of the Caldicott Report and interpretation of the DPA, as related to the practice of medicine, into their practice guidelines 'Confidentiality: Protecting and Providing Information'. These guidelines have been recently updated (April, 2004) and provide a valuable initial reference guide for the clinician.

## FURTHER READING

### Books

Kennedy I and Grubb A. Medical records, and confidentiality. In: *Medical Law*, 3rd edition. Butterworths, London, 2000, Chapters 7 and 8, pp. 990–1047

### Journals

Boyd P. The requirements of the Data Protection Act, 1998 for the processing of medical data. *J Med Ethic* 2003; **29**: 34–35

Case P. Confidence matters: the rise and fall of informational autonomy in Medical Law. *Med Law Rev* 2003; **11**: 208–236

Peto J, Fletcher O and Gilham C. Data protection, informed consent, and research. *Br Med J* 2004; **328**: 1029–1030

### Internet

Access to Health Records Act, 1990. http://www.hmso.gov.uk/acts/acts1990/Ukpga_19900023_en_1.htm#end

Access to Medical Reports Act, 1988. http://www.hmso.gov.uk/acts/acts1988/Ukpga_19880028_en_1.htm

British Medical Association. Access to Health Records by Patients. http://www.bma.org.uk/ap.nsf/Content/accesshealthrecords

British Medical Association. Access to Medical Reports Act 1988. http://www.bma.org.uk/ap.nsf/Content/accessmedreps

British Medical Association. Confidentiality and Disclosure of Health Information. http://www.bma.org.uk/ap.nsf/Content/Confidentiality+and+disclosure+of+health+information

British Medical Association. Guidelines for Doctors receiving Requests from Solicitors to Release Patient Notes for Litigation Purposes.

http://www.bma.org.uk/ap.nsf/Content/Requests+from+solicitors+to+release+
    patient+notes+for+litigation+purposes
British Medical Association. Performing HIV Tests for Life Insurance Companies.
    http://www.bma.org.uk/ap.nsf/Content/Performing+HIV+tests+for+life+
    insurance+companies
Confidentiality: NHS Code of Practice, July 2003. http://www.doh.gov.uk/ipu/confiden
Data Protection Act, 1998. http://www.hmso.gov.uk/acts/acts1998/19980029.htm
Data Protection Act, 1998. Protection and Use of Patient Information.
    http://www.doh.gov.uk/dpa98/
General Medical Council. Serious Communicable Diseases, October, 1997.
    http://www.gmc-uk.org/standards/default.htm
General Medical Council. Confidentiality: Protecting and Providing Information,
    April, 2004. http://www.gmc-uk.org/standards/default.htm
The Caldicott Report, December, 1997. http://www.publications.doh.gov.uk/ipu/
    confiden/report/

## Legal cases

MS v Sweden [1997] 28 EHRR 313
W v Egdell [1990] 1 All ER 835 (CA)
X v Finland [1997] 25 EHRR 371
X v Y [1988] 2 All ER 648

# 8
# Abortion

*'I will not give to a woman an abortive remedy'*

– Hippocratic Oath

The termination of a pregnancy is potentially one of the most difficult and harrowing decisions a woman can make. This process of decision-making has a profound impact on the practice of medicine. Doctors have to be aware of their legal and ethical duties to the patient, even though these may be at odds with their own personal morals or beliefs, and without unnecessarily intruding on the privacy of the patient concerning their decision. In particular the doctor should pay consideration to the fact that it is the patient (and their family) who have to deal with the emotional and personal consequences of their decision.

In 2001, 186,274 terminations were carried out in the UK, 88% because it was considered a risk to the mother's mental or physical health. Eighty-three per cent of terminations were performed before 12 weeks gestational age.

## ETHICS

Abortion has been a contentious issue for many centuries in the UK, although both the level of debate and the politicisation of abortion are not as comprehensive or polarising as in the USA, where potential presidential candidates are expected to make their sentiments known on the subject (and where doctors have been murdered for performing abortions), or in other countries around the world (notably, countries where Islam or Catholicism is the predominant religion).

The abortion issue encompasses a number of different views and value systems. These range from deeply held religious convictions and religious orthodoxy to concerns about the sanctity of human life (and what it means to be human), concerns about the relative personal freedoms of individual women (and whether society has any business determining issues of their autonomy), and concerns about the cost to humanity in terms of poverty and rapid human population expansion.

The traditional basis for the opposition of abortion (and for that matter, contraception) has been founded around the moral and religious 'sanctity of life' principle. Most people consider that it is wrong to kill people. Some people think that killing other humans is wrong in all circumstances ('strict deontology'), while other think that in special circumstances, for example, war or self-defence, killing can be justified ('situational deontology'). However, most people normally think that a special justification is needed when one human kills another, which assumes that the killing is necessary to avoid a greater wrong or evil; for example, an individual might be considered justified in shooting his friend dead if that friend was burning to death in a car crash from which he could not be rescued.

A commonly held view is that some principle of the 'sanctity of life' has to be included in the ultimate principles of any acceptable moral, or functioning social, system. Endorsement of such an absolute principle, however, brings with it a number of contraversial problems:

1  Is all life sacred, or is it just human life? Some animal liberationists, for example, would advocate animal life as being of equal moral worth to human life. By extension, if society considers non-human life as less morally valuable than human life but permits abortion, does that mean that society, on a moral level, equates foetuses with animals?

2  How can society accommodate the sanctity of life principle in situations where there are competing or conflicting interests? In the case of abortion, for example, if we accept that the foetus is a moral being whose life is sacrosanct, should it always be the case that the mother should risk sacrificing her own life to avoid the risk of killing her foetus?

3  Where does the boundary between life and death actually lie – when does human life begin? Is a human embryo alive in the same sense as a foetus, or is a foetus alive in the same sense as a child? Is the concept of life absolute (i.e. does the foetus become 'alive' after a defined point), or is it a graded concept (i.e. does the foetus gradually become more alive during intrauterine development)? Furthermore, what is the role of 'potentiality' in the debate – does the potential of an embryo to become a human carry the same moral worth as being recognisably human? If society were to accept that an embryo is alive or has the potential to become alive, are sperm or eggs also 'alive' and therefore owed protection according to any

sanctity of life principle (thus making contraception, and artificial reproduction technologies, morally dubious)?

4 Is being alive intrinsically valuable? Is the life of a severely brain-damaged and disabled child born prematurely at 24 weeks gestation of any intrinsic value or worth to that child or its family if by being alive that child and their family endure considerable physical and mental suffering. Furthermore, is it the case that some lives are not worth living? If this is the case, then is it also the case that society can determine which lives are worth living, or is this uncomfortably close to an endorsement of negative eugenics? Should decisions about the worthiness of life be left to those who bear the burdens and impact of having children? Should society impose any limits on these decisions about worthiness made by individuals?

5 Is being alive the same as being a person? What are the specific characteristics of human beings that elevate the species above mere existence? Are foetuses of less moral worth because they may lack these characteristics? By extension, is the killing of infants, the permanently unconscious and the severely mentally ill morally justified on the basis that these groups may also lack these characteristics? Again, what is the role of potentiality in the debate, and where does it leave the moral value of the severely brain-damaged premature baby?

The authors apologise for not making any effort to answer these questions. However, it may be that there are no convincing or conclusive answers, which illustrates the reason why the abortion debate is so divisive.

Temporally, abortion is the destruction of life after conception and before birth. It is bounded by non-fertilisation of the egg at one extreme, and by infanticide at the other. The questions that arise are:

- When it might be morally acceptable to perform an abortion?
- Are there any ethical principles that can guide the practitioner?

Abortion is defended by some on the basis that the embryo and early foetus are very distinct from fully formed human beings to the extent that there is little difference between contraception and abortion in the early stages of pregnancy. They also point out that foetuses are often aborted naturally in any case (it is estimated that a third of confirmed pregnancies spontaneously abort before 8 weeks gestation, and are incapable of independent life). In contrast, anti-abortionists ('prolifers') tend to focus on the 'rights' of the unborn child as a human being, and stress the problems in distinguishing between abortion and infanticide.

Both of these arguments promote the idea that there is a definable point at which human life becomes recognisable (and therefore morally valid). For pro-abortionists, this point is birth itself (such that the foetus may be aborted at any point during gestation); for anti-abortionists, this point is around the time of conception. Pragmatically, in the UK a compromise point of 24 weeks is used, because this is seen currently as the point before which premature birth is unsurvivable despite medical intervention (Figure 8.1).

Both utilitarianism and deontology can accommodate the notion of abortion. Abortion is viewed as morally acceptable (or, at least, not morally wrong) by utilitarianism if it maximises happiness: this may be the case, for example, if the happiness of the mother in having an abortion (retained autonomy, inability to cope socially, physically or mentally with damaged foetus) outweighed the negative consequences (sanctity of life arguments, effects of abortion on society, etc.). Further 'happiness' might accrue if the calculation were to start with the precept that the foetus is not a human being, and has an uncertain potential to become a human being. The deontological position is less certain, and involves the resolution of a conflict of duties, namely 'not killing' and 'respecting autonomy'. Again greater credence may be given to 'respecting autonomy' if it is accepted that the foetus is not/is less of a moral entity than a human being, although conversely, deontological arguments (or for that matter religious beliefs) may be used by an individual to derogate from their personal involvement in performing abortions.

The problem with utilitarianism and deontology is that it is difficult to apply them to the emotive and complex ethical dilemmas surrounding the everyday practice of abortion. More commonly, a 'rights'-based approach is used. Foremost in the case of abortion is the right of a pregnant woman to self-determination, embodied in the right of a woman to choose whether or not to have an abortion (the 'feminist perspective'). Several arguments have been advanced in support of this position, including:

- Abortion as self-defence against an invader. This formed one of the pillars of the argument developed by Judith Jarvis Thomson in her seminal paper 'A defense of abortion', in which she argued that, although the foetus can be considered a person from the moment of conception, the mother is entitled to defend her life against the threat to it posed by the unborn child, even if doing so involves the death of the child. However, this rationale only supports abortion if the life of the mother is in danger.
- The notion of priority of the mother's rights over any putative rights of the unborn foetus. Thomson uses an intriguing analogy to

| Time after conception | Prolife position | Prochoice position |
|---|---|---|
| | Argument against termination at this time | Argument in favour of termination at this time |
| Preconception | Contraception may prevent the creation of a potential person | • Contraception is a right<br>• No 'potential person' has even been created |
| Conception | The foetus is a potential person | A third of all foetuses at this stage are naturally aborted, therefore potentiality is not an issue |
| 6–7 weeks: consciousness | The foetus is moving and may be able to feel pain, and therefore is a sentient being | Sentience is not the same as consciousness |
| 12–18 weeks: quickening | Movements are felt, and may be responsive to maternal activity for example, eating. Reactivity indicates thought and increased consciousness | Reactivity may be reflex rather than subjectively controlled |
| 24 weeks: viability | • Premature infants are able to survive after this time, albeit with medical assistance<br>• Medical technology, including intrauterine surgery, is likely to consistently improve the meaningful survival of barely viable foetuses | • Barely viable foetuses born at this time have a minimal chance of a meaningful survival<br>• A number of inherited conditions may be present that are incompatible with foetal/early infant survival |
| 36 weeks: survivable prematurity | Although premature, foetuses should survive unaided after this time | • A number of inherited or obstetric conditions may be present that are incompatible with foetal/early infant survival<br>• The mothers life (and, by extension, continued foetal existence may be at risk through continuation of the pregnancy |
| 40 weeks: birth | The location (i.e. *in utero/ ex utero*) of what is, to all intents and purposes, a baby should make no difference – it is wrong to kill a baby, therefore, it is wrong to kill a term foetus | • A number of inherited or obstetric conditions may be present that are incompatible with foetal/early infant survival<br>• The mothers life (and, by extension, continued foetal existence may be at risk through continuation of the pregnancy |
| In general | • The preservation of life is sacrosanct<br>• The foetus is a potential human<br>• Society cares for other individuals with 'no meaningful life' (the demented, those with Persistent Vegetative State (PVS)) | • Foetal life has limited, if any, value<br>• Foetal life has limited value in comparison to a woman's right to autonomous action |

**Figure 8.1** Arguments for and against abortion at various stages of gestation.

support this position. She asks the reader to imagine that they wake up one morning to find themselves surgically attached to an unconscious person. The person turns out to be a famous violinist, suffering from a fatal kidney ailment. A Society of Music Lovers has kidnapped the reader, attached the violinist, and now tells the reader that the violinist will remain attached for 9 months until he recovers, pointing out that to detach the violinist will result in his death. Far from suggesting that the reader would be obliged to carry on providing life support for the violinist, Thomson suggests that the reader would be well within their rights to detach themselves, even if the death of the violinist resulted. By extending the analogy, Thomson implies that similarly, a woman has more of a right to abort a foetus, than a foetus has a right to be born.

Fundamentally, rights-based arguments recognise that it is not necessarily right to kill a foetus, but nevertheless a woman is not obliged to give birth to a child if she chooses not to. In other words, if it were possible to extract a living foetus and raise it artificially by other means, then the rights argument would embody this concept. In practice, there must be another justification for killing the foetus, which is the current legal position: although the primary decision-making is made by the woman as to whether or not to have an abortion, endorsement of this decision is made by the medical profession acting under strict guidance. Endorsement is justified not by moral argument, but by pragmatic assessment of the impact of the pregnancy on the rights and interests of the mother, and others, in comparison to any rights that the foetus might have. It is incumbent on the medical profession to assess the balance of harms to various individuals when endorsing the decision by a mother to have an abortion.

## LAW

An unlawful abortion (namely, 'procuring a miscarriage') is a crime that can be committed by either the pregnant woman or others under Sections 58 and 59 of the Offences against the Person Act, 1861 (OAPA). These sections were not included to outlaw abortion *per se*, but rather aimed at protecting women from unscrupulous and unsafe doctors and their practices.

Conversely, the common law has developed to allow for medical abortions. In *R v Bourne* [1939] 1B 687, it was held that an abortion would not be unlawful if it was done in good faith for the purpose of preserving the life of the mother. The effect of the impact on the mother was expanded to include both her mental and physical health (*R v Bergmann* [1948] 1 *BMJ* 1008, *R v Newron and Stungo* [1958] Crim LR 469). However, a degree of confusion and concern remained in the common law as to the parameters defining the lawfulness of providing an abortion. This was resolved by the passing of the Abortion Act, 1967 (subsequently modified by the Abortion Regulations, 1991). The Abortion Act provides for a statutory defence to Sections 58 and 59 of the OAPA, providing two medical practitioners, acting in good faith, are satisfied that:

- Section 1(1)(a) – there is a risk of physical or mental injury to the mother, namely that 'the risk of continuing pregnancy is greater than risk of termination'. This is the cause given for 97% of UK abortions. The abortion must be performed within 24 weeks of the first day of the patient's last menstruation.
- Section 1(1)(b) – termination would 'prevent grave permanent injury to the physical or mental health of the mother'. This section was introduced by 1991 amendments. No question of relative risk is involved, only the question of whether termination is 'necessary', for example, in cases involving severe pregnancy-induced hypertension, breast or cervical cancer, or suicidal women. Termination may be carried out later than 24 weeks after the first day of the patient's last menstruation.
- Section 1(1)(c) – there is a risk to the life of the mother. Termination must 'reduce the risk to the mother's life, rather than remove the risk', for example, by reducing the cardiovascular stress associated with pregnancy continuation in women with underlying heart disease.
- Section 1(1)(d) – there is 'substantial risk that the child may be seriously handicapped'. In this case, the risk of severe handicap must be more probable than not, and includes serious defects rather than just undesirable ones. Termination may be carried out later than 24 weeks after the first day of the patient's last menstruation.

It should be noted that, until the 1991 regulations came into force, the Abortion Act had to be understood with reference to the effect of the Infant Life (Preservation) Act, 1929 (ILPA). Under these circumstances, compliance with the Abortion Act did not provide a defence to the crime of child destruction' created by the ILPA. The ILPA was created to close a gap in the law, whereby a child could be killed in the course of being born, which was neither an offence under Section 58 of the OAPA (i.e. not a miscarriage), nor was it murder or manslaughter as there was no independence from the mother. Aborting a foetus 'capable of being born alive' under the ILPA amounted to a criminal offence. Although there was no precise definition in statutory law, until 1991 the upper time limit for a legal abortion was somewhere between 22 and 24 weeks gestation, depending on the development of the foetus. Now terminations may not be carried out after 24 weeks, except when the child may be seriously handicapped.

The primary ground for abortion (Section 1(1)(a) Abortion Act) requires that the certifying doctors engage in a comparative exercise and decide whether there is a greater risk to the mother's (or existing children's) physical or mental health if the pregnancy continued, rather than if it were terminated. It is not sufficient that the pregnancy creates a risk to the mother's or existing children's physical or mental health. The 'risk' to the pregnant woman is very broad in its definition. Many of the terminations performed under this ground have been classified as 'social abortions' because the pregnancy is unwanted, or is an inconvenience to the mother and her family. Nevertheless, it is a truism that the doctors must always be satisfied of the effect on the mother's health. However, distress and mental well-being can encompass all of the deleterious effects on a woman's life. The doctors do not have to be satisfied that this effect is certain or probable but rather there is a 'greater risk'. In assessing the impact on the woman, account must be taken of her actual or foreseeable environment. Risk assessment should take into account the quality and extent of medical and social evidence, and should not focus merely on the risks manifest at the point in time when the decision to terminate is taken. Doctors are also asked to examine the impact of the completion of the pregnancy on existing children. In the act, the definition of a child is not limited to the standard legal definition of 'under 18', and can contemplate the impact on adult children.

Section 1(1)(b) introduced a new substantive ground for obtaining an abortion. Prior to amendment by the Abortion Regulations 1991, Section 1(1)(b) had merely justified carrying out an abortion in an National Health Service (NHS) hospital or approved clinic. There is no time limit on Section 1(1)(b); consistent with the remaining grounds, Parliament did not seek to impose a time limit on abortions when serious dangers to a woman's health existed. Section 1(1)(b) requires an injury of a different order of magnitude to Section 1(1)(a), requiring manifest proof of a specified danger. On the face of it, the comparative exercise in Section 1(1)(a) is abandoned. The termination must be 'necessary' to avoid some or all of the specified injury, as opposed to reducing the 'risk' of 'grave injury'. The injury under Section 1(1)(b) must be actual or certain to occur; when this is not the case, doctors will have to rely on Section 1(1)(a) as a default with the 24-week time limit now operative. Section 1(1)(b) only applies where termination is effectively a last resort.

Prior to implementation of the Abortion Regulations 1991, the ground in Section 1(1)(c), 'Risk to woman's life', was embodied in what is now Section 1(1)(a). Section 1(1)(c) also requires two certifying doctors to engage in the comparative assessment of risks, but concentrates on the risk to the mother's life. The law only requires that the termination reduces the risk to the mother's life, rather than eliminating the risk to life altogether. There may be a continuing but lesser risk, but the termination will fall within Section 1(1)(c) if she stands a better chance of survival after having the termination. This consideration may be important in respect of selective reduction procedures where one or more foetuses are terminated *in utero* when the woman has a multiple pregnancy.

Lawful termination under the final ground, Section 1(1)(d), may be satisfied if two doctors were of the opinion that there is a substantial risk that, if the child were to be born, it would be seriously handicapped due to physical or mental abnormalities. The interpretation of this ground is not without some problems. In theory, a termination could be obtained under this ground after the foetus is 24 weeks old. Although there can be a few foetal abnormalities that are detected late in pregnancy, there is a general trend that terminations are performed earlier rather than later. Also, many gynaecologists are reluctant to perform a termination late in pregnancy, on the ground that the foetus is seriously handicapped, unless the disablement is unusually severe, for example, in ancephaly, a condition in which most of the foetal cerebral cortex is missing. However, some difficulties remain with the interpretation and application of this ground. It is unclear what is meant by a 'substantial risk' in this context. This is compounded by the requirement that the doctor need only have an 'honest belief' that the risk is substantial. For example, if a mistake of fact is made as to the risk (i.e. that it was thought the risk was 50% when it was only 25%) then good faith ('honest belief') will provide a defence in law. However, if the mistake is not factual but rather an assessment of whether the 25% risk was substantial, good faith will not provide a defence if a judge takes the view that this was a misinterpretation of the ground in the act. Nevertheless, it is likely that the courts will tend to give any doctors exercising this ground the benefit of the doubt.

The phrase 'seriously handicapped' also presents problems. An assessment by medical experts is required, and the definition is not limited to children who are 'grossly abnormal and unable to lead any meaningful life' (See House of Lords Select Committee report on Infant Life (Preservation) Bill, 1987–1988 No. 50, p. 18). The major concern here is an assessment of the parents' ability to cope with a seriously disabled child.

In practice, less serious conditions form the ground for abortion under this section. Providing that the condition is not trivial (e.g. easily treated conditions such as cleft palate), the law allows doctors wide scope in the application of this section. Most serious genetic or biochemical conditions that manifest themselves at birth, or shortly after, fall under the ambit of this ground. The question that remains concerns *when* the condition manifests itself. Huntingdon's disease, for example, is an inherited disease which may take many years to affect an individual such that their quality of life becomes subjectively intolerable (if at all). The solution relies on an interpretation of the meaning of 'child' in this context, as the statute seems concerned with the impact of the disorder in childhood.

Terminations may take place in NHS hospitals (NHS Act, 1977) (NHS hospitals are the only places in which terminations may be carried out later than 24 weeks), private clinics (with the approval of the Secretary of State for Health) and by general practitioners (GPs) (in the case of the morning after pill).

The Abortion Act requires that the opinion of two doctors must be given in the prescribed form of the 'certificate of opinion', set out Schedule 1, Part 1 of the 1991 Regulations. No other form of certification is permissible. The Regulations also provide that the doctor performing the termination has to notify the appropriate Chief Medical Officer of the termination. The doctor performing the termination does not have to be the same one who certified.

Doctors may conscientiously object to taking part in terminations (Section 4(1) of the Abortion Act), provided that they can prove their objection, and the life of the mother is not at risk or that she is at risk of suffering grave, permanent injury. However, the obligation remains to advise the patient, and to refer her to another medical practitioner who is prepared to provide the service for her (see *R v Salford Health Authority, ex parte Janaway* [1989] AC 537).

Fathers and others have no standing in law to prevent terminations (fathers as fathers: *Paton v Trustees of BPAS* [1979] QB 276; fathers as next friends of the unborn child: *St Georges Healthcare NHS Trust v S, R v Collins, ex parte S* [1998] 44 BMLR 160 (CA); fathers as protectors of the public interest: *Paton v Trustees of BPAS* [1979] QB 276), or even be consulted about a proposed termination. The human rights aspects of terminations (i.e. right to life under Article 2, and right to respect for private and family life under Article 8) were considered in *Paton v UK* [1980] 3 EHRR 408 (EComHR), which found current UK law to be in line with the European Convention on Human Rights (and therefore, subsequently, the Human Rights Act 1998, (HRA). Nevertheless, this issue may be revisited given the enactment of the HRA and the limited application of *Paton* to early abortions. It may be the case that termination under Sections 1(1)(b)–(d) may be the subject of challenge under the HRA, in future.

## Selective reductions

Section 5(2) of the Abortion Act, 1967, has been amended by the Human Fertilisation and Embryology Act, 1990. The effect of this provision is to bring the two procedures of selective reduction and selective foeticide within the Abortion Act. Section 5(2) assumes that these procedures do not procure a miscarriage for the purposes of the OAPA. Section 5(2)(a) covers procedures for selective foeticide where a particular foetus is selected by pre-natal screening. Provided the foetus could be aborted on the grounds of foetal abnormality, then that foetus alone can be terminated as part of a multiple pregnancy. Section 5(2)(a) covers selective reduction techniques. If the doctor is satisfied that termination is necessary under Section 1(1) of the Abortion Act, they may reduce the number of foetuses in a pregnancy in order to reduce the risk to the life of the mother. Section 5(2)(b) does not require the doctor to specifically identify a disabled foetus, and allows random selection of a foetus. It is worth noting, however, that although selective reduction may also reduce the risk to other foetuses, Section 5(2) does not provide this as a ground for termination under Section 1(1) of the Abortion Act, only a risk to the mother will satisfy this ground.

## Counselling

Prior to undergoing elective termination of pregnancy, it is obligatory for mothers to undergo some form of counselling or advice prior to the procedure. In practice, such counselling is provided by doctors prior to obtaining consent for the procedure. It is vital in these circumstances that the form of advice and counselling remain value neutral, so that the decision-making of the mother is informed and voluntary.

## FURTHER READING

### Books

Glover J. *Causing Death and Saving Lives*. Penguin, London, 1977, Chapters 3, 9–12

Kennedy and Grubb (Eds). Abortion. In: *Medical Law*, 3rd edition. Butterworths, London, 2000, Chapter 11, pp. 1405–1492

## Journals

Greenwood M. The new ethics of abortion. *J Med Ethic* 2001; **27**: 2ii–4
Marquis D. Why abortion is wrong. *J Philos* 1989; **86**: 183–202
Thomson JJ. A defense of abortion. *Philos Public Aff* 1971; **1**: 47–66
Wicclair MR. Conscientious objection in medicine. *Bioethics* 2000; **14**: 205–227

## Internet

Abortion statistics. Office for National Statistics.
    http://www.statistics.gov.uk/CCI/nscl.asp?ID=6249
British Medical Association. *The Law and Ethics of Abortion*.
    http://www.bma.org.uk/ap.nsf/Content/abortion
ProLife Alliance. http://www.prolife.org.uk/

# 9

# Products liability

The field of products liability is a large and specialised area of legal practise. In the context of perioperative medicine, products liability is concerned with the following questions:

1 Who is liable when a faulty product is alleged to have caused harm to a patient?
2 Can a defendant in a case of negligence claim that faulty equipment contributed to the harm caused to a patient?

## ETHICS

In spite of developments in the law to protect consumers against negligence, highly publicised cases arising from the use of defective products (e.g. silicon breast implants, Bjork–Shiley heart valves) have brought pressure on successive governments to reform the law concerning products liability.

A key turning point came with the Thalidomide tragedy of the late 1950s and early 1960s. Thalidomide was marketed as a treatment for morning sickness in pregnant women, but hundreds of babies worldwide were born with varying degrees of phocomelia or abnormally developed limbs, as an unforeseen side effect of the drug. As the tort of negligence relies on demonstrating fault and foreseeable harm, it was very difficult for claimants at the time to recover damages against manufacturers. Naturally, these events gave rise to considerable public concern. There was an understandable perception that a great injustice had been perpetrated in these circumstances, without any possibility of the injustice being righted or prevented by the law. As a result, Thalidomide had its product licence withdrawn (it may still be prescribed in the UK on a named patient basis – and indeed appears to be making something of a comeback as an anti-inflammatory drug), and the matter prompted re-examination of the law of products liability by legal reformers.

It should be remembered that not all harms relating to faulty products are foreseeable. Companies may not, in fact, be negligent or blameworthy in the development of their product – human error, either in incorrect administration of a drug or the imprecise use of equipment, is often contributory. Nevertheless, considerable harm may have occurred to the patient through use of the product.

Eventually, change in the law was accomplished as part of European Community (EC) law. A 'Product Liability' Directive (85/374/EEC) was adopted in 1985, which obliged the UK to create domestic legislation incorporating the provisions of the directive. This was achieved by Part I of the Consumer Protection Act, 1987 (CPA).

The aims of this new statutory regime are identified by reciting that part of the directive which states that '[L]iability without fault on the part of the producer is the only way of solving the problem, peculiar to our age of increasing technicality, of a fair apportionment of the risks inherent in modern technological production'. However, the European Court of Justice has ruled that Article 94 of the EC treaty, which provides for harmonisation of the laws of the EC, prevents individual Member States from implementing more stringent forms of liability than established by the Directive (or even maintaining existing national provisions that give greater consumer protection than under the Directive), the perception being that differences in consumer protection in different member states might distort competition, and impede the free movement of goods. The EEC recognise that there is considerable commercial investment by companies in the development of a new product, and that the profitability of new products allows these companies to develop further treatments. However, it is also recognised that member states have a duty to protect their citizens from harm – in this case, the marketing and use of products with an adverse risk/benefit ratio.

However, it is arguable that political and commercial considerations, to some extent, appear consistently to trump any moral imperatives that might afford consumers more effective protection against dangerous medical products, the exception being if large numbers of people are affected, or if possible claims in negligence are likely to be expensive.

Some sceptics have suggested that, in terms of consumer protection, the statutory scheme is flawed as it is no easier to prove that a product is defective than to prove that it was negligently manufactured. Other commentators have suggested that the statutory scheme provides speedier and cheaper remedies thus benefiting consumers. In any case in Britain the statutory remedies operate alongside existing remedies in contract and tort.

## LAW

In terms of medical law, products liability is concerned with medicinal products (i.e. drugs) and medical devices. Liability claims may follow injury caused by either type, and may be based in contract or negligence, or under the CPA.

Actions in contract do not arise under contract law, because patients do not form contracts with hospitals or doctors when receiving NHS care; contract law may be used in cases involving private hospitals or doctors, however, when these act as suppliers of medical care.

## Contract

In the law of contract, claimant consumers can exercise very powerful rights against defendants if they can establish that a contract had been formed between the contracting parties. Contractual remedies are available even when the defendant is in no way at 'fault', as liability for breach of contract is, in general, strict. Moreover, the common law of contract is supported by the Sale of Goods Act, 1979 which implies terms into contracts of sale such that goods are of a satisfactory quality and reasonably fit for their purpose. However, these rights are directly limited to the purchaser of the goods under the contract.

## Negligence

The most famous products liability case is, perhaps, one of the most famous cases in tort law. It is arguable that no defective product has ever achieved the fame of the rotting snail in Mrs Donoghue's bottle of ginger beer (*Donoghue v Stevenson* [1932] AC 562). For the first time, this case accepted that consumers had rights against the manufacturers of defective products in the tort of negligence that they lacked under the law of contract.

The development of the law in negligence serves the interests of consumers well. Although in theory the burden of establishing 'fault' falls on the consumer, in practice the presence of a defect in the product gives rise to an inference of negligence on the part of the manufacturer (*Grant v Australian Knitting Mills* [1936] AC 85).

Claims in negligence require the plaintiff to prove that a breach of duty on the part of the manufacturer caused the injury sustained by the patient, when the product failed. The duty owed by the manufacturer depends on the product:

- the manufacture, marketing and sale of medicinal products are regulated by the Medicines Act, 1968;

- since June, 1998, the safety and performance of all medical devices must comply with the Medical Devices Directive (93/42/EEC) and enforcement of the Medical Devices Regulations, 1994.

In general, the manufacturers may be liable for manufacturing defects, design defects, marketing defects (e.g. 'failure to warn') and post-marketing defects (i.e. manufacturers have a continuing duty of care).

## The Consumer Protection Act, 1987

The CPA requires manufacturers to carry the risk of their products causing injury (i.e. 'strict' liability, as opposed to 'fault based' liability, which is similar to no fault compensation after medical errors) and therefore provide compensation to injured parties.

The basic definition of a 'product' is found in Section 1(2) of the act. It includes products that comprise component parts of larger products, as well as the raw materials from which they are made. An issue arises as to whether information contained in books or computer programs amounts to a product for the purposes of the act. A number of commentators have suggested that these cases are outside the scope of the act, as information is not, of itself, a product and does not become a product even when incorporated into a book. However, the contrary view is that a book itself can be regarded as a product, whose defectiveness results from the unsafe information it contains. For example, an operating manual that incorrectly provides information on how to use a cystoscope, such that a potentially avoidable perforation of the bladder results, may or may not be considered to be a faulty product.

The act does not hold the producer liable for all the harm caused by their products. The producer may only be liable if their product is 'defective'. The liability under this act is one of 'defect liability' rather than 'strict liability' that is, the company that sells the defective product is only liable for injury that results from the defective product, rather than for all injuries that may occur after the use of a defective product. The test for defectiveness is found in Section 3(1), such that

> 'there is a defect in a product ... if the safety of the product is not such as persons are generally entitled to expect'

Note that the test refers to the safety of the product, not its usefulness. For products that simply do not work a claimant has to find a remedy via contract. Also, the test is framed in terms of public expectation, rather than whether the manufacturer has exercised reasonable care and skill (which is the test in negligence). The court must consider what the public are entitled to expect, which is a test of legitimate expectation rather than actual expectation, such that the public are entitled to expect product safety in line with what information about the product is in the public domain. Once the public have been educated about the risks associated with a product, their expectations may be reduced. For example, in *A and Others v National Blood Authority and Another* [2001] 3 All ER 289, a group-action case which considered whether the defendants were liable for injury under the CPA resulting from Hepatitis C contamination of blood transfusions, the judge found that at the relevant time there was no public understanding or acceptance of the infection of transfused blood, but concluded that the public were entitled to expect the blood to be safe and uninfected.

What consumers are entitled to expect about the safety of a product depends on 'all the circumstances (being) taken into account' (Section 3(2) of the act). This includes, for example, marketing and presentation, such that the way in which a product is advertised could affect the legitimate expectation of the consumer. There is also a requirement regarding any warnings or instructions on the product. For example, many drugs are lethal if taken in large quantities, but would not be regarded as defective if the correct dose was clearly stated and an appropriate warning against exceeding the specified dose was prominently displayed. Steps taken to convey the warning need only be proportionate to the risk.

However, the CPA does not impose absolute liability, and manufacturers can defend themselves on the basis of 'development risks', such that liability is escaped if the manufacturer can prove that the state of scientific and technical knowledge at the time when he put the product into circulation was not such as to enable the existence of a defect to be discovered (Section 4) (the 'state of the art' defence). As yet there is a paucity of case law, the leading judgement being the decision in *A and Others v National Blood Authority and Another* [2001] 3 All ER 289 (see above), when the High Court rejected the defendant's claim of 'development risks' as a defence against damages.

The CPA confers a right to sue on any person who suffers damage from a defective product. Most forms of damage are covered apart from damage to the product itself or for pure economic loss. Primary liability is imposed on the 'producer', 'own brander' and any importer of the product into the European Union (EU) who supplies another business. The application of the CPA to the production and supply of medical products is far reaching. Any person in the chain of supply of the product can be liable if they fail, on request, to identify their supplier or the producer within a reasonable time frame, or when reasonably practicable.

If a claimant can prove that damage has been caused by a defective product for which any of the above defendants is responsible under the

CPA, the burden of proof shifts to the defendants to prove that any of the six defences listed in Section 4 of the act applies:

- Section 4(1)(a) that the defect is attributable to compliance with any requirement imposed by or under any enactment or with any Community EU obligation. Of itself, mere compliance is not enough. The defendant must show that the compliance caused the defect, for example, compliance with the licensing regulations under the Medicines Act 1968 is not a defence although it will be of evidential value in relation to consumer expectations and development risks. The requirement relied on must be mandatory:
- Sections 4(1)(b) and 46 require that the defendant did not at anytime supply the product to another. This is relied on where damage has arisen from the theft of drugs or from the use of defective products provided that they are not yet in the distribution chain.
- Section 4(1)(c) requires that the defendant did not supply the drugs in the course of their business or with a producer, importer or own brander with a view to a profit.
- Sections 4(1)(d) and 4(2) require that the defect did not exist in the product at the relevant time. This could arise when drugs are inadequately stored leading them to deteriorate, or are tampered with.
- Section 4(1)(e) covers the 'development risks defence'. This requires that the state of scientific and technical knowledge at the relevant time was not such that the producer of products of the same description as the product in question might have been expected to discover the defect in their product while it was under their control. This is one of the most controversial aspects of the legislation as it was heavily lobbied for by the pharmaceutical industry to protect innovation and insurability. It has been criticised on the ground that it merely reverts the scheme of the act to tests of negligence. The controversy has been exacerbated by the difference in the terminology in the CPA compared to the equivalent provision (Article 7(e)) in the EU directive. The directive requires that the defendant prove that the state of knowledge 'was not such as to enable the existence of the defect to be discovered', and is concerned with what is objectively discoverable, whereas the CPA is concerned with what might be expected of producers of a particular category of products to discover.
- Section 4(1)(f) requires that the defect in the component is wholly attributable to the design of the finished product in which it was comprised or to compliance with the instructions of that manufacturer.

In general, normal periods of limitation apply under the CPA, apart from limiting personal injury to occurring within 3 years of exposure to the defective product, and setting an upper limit of 10 years in bringing a claim. Group or class actions, where a number of claimants join together in taking a company to court, are now acceptable.

## Medicines and Healthcare Products Regulatory Agency

The Medicines and Healthcare Products Regulatory Agency (MHRA) is a government organisation, similar to those found in other countries, set up with the aim of ensuring that medicines and medical equipment in the UK meet appropriate standards of safety, quality and efficacy, in order to safeguard public health. 'Safety' covers potential or actual harmful effects, 'quality' relates to development and manufacture, and 'efficacy' is a measure of the beneficial effect of the medicine on patients. The Medicines Control Agency and the Medical Devices Agency have been incorporated into this new body.

The aims of the MHRA are achieved in a number of ways, including:

- provision of a system of licensing before the marketing of medicines;
- monitoring of medicines and acting on safety concerns after they have been placed on the market;
- checking standards of pharmaceutical manufacture and wholesaling;
- provision of a device evaluation service;
- enforcement of requirements and regulations;
- responsibility for medicines control policy;
- representing UK pharmaceutical regulatory interests internationally;
- publishing quality standards for drug substances through the British Pharmacopoeia.

## FURTHER READING

### Book

Kennedy and Grubb (Eds). Products liability. In: *Medical Law*, 3rd edition. Chapters 13, pp. 1594–1664

### Journals

Commentary. Consumer Protection Act, 1987: liability for defective products. *Med Law Rev* 2002; **10**: 82–88

Dimond B. The relevance of the Consumer Protection Act, 1987 to health care. *Br J Nurs* 2002; **11**: 1068–1070

Hodges C. The reuse of medical devices. *Med Law Rev* 2000; **8**: 157–181

## Internet

Medical Devices Agency. http://www.medical-devices.gov.uk/

Medicines and Healthcare Products Regulatory Agency. http://www.mca.gov.uk/

# 10

# Research

*'Medical progress is based on research which ultimately must rest in part on experimentation involving human subjects.'*
— Principle 4, Declaration of Helsinki
(World Medical Association)

All interventional medical treatment has resulted from research. Future cures or improvements in medical therapy rely on continued research, and this necessarily must include research performed on human beings. Observational research is without the remit of the law. Interventional research, however, is prescribed by rigid sets of ethical and practical guidelines (failure to comply with which is viewed poorly by the courts), and common law, particularly in relation to consent and medical negligence.

## ETHICS

The quest for medical knowledge has not always been carried out in the most ethical of fashions. In the 1st century BC, for example, Cleopatra is reputed to have had a number of her handmaidens impregnated, and subsequently operated upon at certain times of gestation, in order to test the theory that it took 40 days for a male foetus to form, compared to 80 days for a female foetus. In 1796, Edward Jenner injected a healthy 8-year-old boy, James Phillips, with cowpox, then 3 months later with smallpox, in order to prove that the former provided defence against the latter. Between about 1850 and 1980, there are numerous documented reports of doctors in the US using soldiers, prisoners, orphans and others as subjects in research trials of dubious validity and value. From 1932 to 1945, the Japanese subjected tens of thousands of captured Chinese subjects to a number of horrifying experiments, some of which involved live vivisection.

However, much of current ethical opinion concerning research on human subjects was formed in the light of the barbarism of Nazi doctors in the Second World War, as recounted by military prosecutors at the

Nuremberg trials, in 1945. Summing up, Judges Beals, Sebring and Crawford stated 10 principles (the Nuremberg code – Figure 10.1) that should always inform ethical human experimentation, including the absolute requirement for patient consent, and the requirement for doctors to put the welfare of the study subject before the necessity for the research.

The Nuremberg code was supplemented by the Declaration of Helsinki (Ethical Principles for Medical Research Involving Human Subjects) of the World Medical Association in 1964 (last amended 2000), which prescribes the basis for ethical human experimentation. This is a comprehensive document, and informs the ethical basis for experimentation both on an international level, and as incorporated into the practice guidelines issued by many national medical bodies (including the General Medical Council (GMC)).

Guidelines concerning human experimentation vary according to whether the research involves:

- Therapeutic or non-therapeutic interventions. Therapeutic research is usually carried out as an adjunct to the medical management of ill patients who might possibly gain from treatment; non-therapeutic research is often carried out on healthy volunteers, for the purposes of gaining knowledge.
- Patients or volunteers.
- Competent or incompetent patients.
- Innovative or pre-existing interventions.

The major ethical principles identified in Chapter 3 underpin the conduct of ethically acceptable research.

## (a) Respect for autonomy

The involvement of competent patients in research should be entirely of their own volition. Similarly, participants must be allowed to withdraw their consent at any time and for any reason. The three recognised components of consent are of fundamental importance:

- *Voluntariness*: This is seldom an issue when patients consent to a medical procedure, as if the procedure is indicated, the patient is invariably happy, or at least co-operative, because the best of advice indicates that their medical condition will improve (or at least not worsen) through treatment. However, there is a measure of altruism involved in participating in research. It is expected that a proposed treatment will work, but often there are no guarantees, and the

1 The voluntary consent of the human subject is absolutely essential. This means that the person involved should have legal capacity to give consent; should be so situated as to be able to exercise free power of choice, without the intervention of any element of force, fraud, deceit, duress, over-reaching, or other ulterior form of constraint or coercion; and should have sufficient knowledge and comprehension of the elements of the subject matter involved as to enable him to make an understanding and enlightened decision. This latter element requires that before the acceptance of an affirmative decision by the experimental subject there should be made known to him the nature, duration, and purpose of the experiment; the method and means by which it is to be conducted; all inconveniences and hazards reasonable to be expected; and the effects upon his health or person which may possibly come from his participation in the experiment.

   The duty and responsibility for ascertaining the quality of the consent rests upon each individual who initiates, directs or engages in the experiment. It is a personal duty and responsibility which may not be delegated to another with impunity.

2 The experiment should be such as to yield fruitful results for the good of society, unprocurable by other methods or means of study, and not random and unnecessary in nature.

3 The experiment should be so designed and based on the results of animal experimentation and a knowledge of the natural history of the disease or other problem under study that the anticipated results will justify the performance of the experiment.

4 The experiment should be so conducted as to avoid all unnecessary physical and mental suffering and injury.

5 No experiment should be conducted where there is an a priori reason to believe that death or disabling injury will occur; except, perhaps, in those experiments where the experimental physicians also serve as subjects.

6 The degree of risk to be taken should never exceed that determined by the humanitarian importance of the problem to be solved by the experiment.

7 Proper preparations should be made and adequate facilities provided to protect the experimental subject against even remote possibilities of injury, disability, or death.

8 The experiment should be conducted only by scientifically qualified persons. The highest degree of skill and care should be required through all stages of the experiment of those who conduct or engage in the experiment.

9 During the course of the experiment the human subject should be at liberty to bring the experiment to an end if he has reached the physical or mental state where continuation of the experiment seems to him to be impossible.

10 During the course of the experiment the scientist in charge must be prepared to terminate the experiment at any stage, if he has probable cause to believe, in the exercise of the good faith, superior skill and careful judgment required of him that a continuation of the experiment is likely to result in injury, disability, or death to the experimental subject.

**Figure 10.1** The Nuremberg code.

subject may in fact be harmed through participation. Therefore, a system of incentives may be advanced in order to facilitate the acquisition of sufficient subject numbers. This may involve an understanding on the part of the subject that participation could in fact improve their medical condition, or financial remuneration for the research subject. The GMC offers the following guidance on financial remuneration:

'You must be open and honest in all financial and commercial matters relating to your research and its funding. In particular you must:

- give participants information on how the research is funded, including any benefits which will accrue to researchers and/or their departments;
- respond honestly and fully to participants' questions, including inquiries about direct payments made to you and any financial interests you have in the research project or its sponsoring organisations;
- not offer payments at a level which could induce research participants to take risks that they would otherwise not take, or to volunteer more frequently than is advisable or against their better interests or judgment.'

Some critics have argued that, in terms of autonomy, it is surely the decision of the subjects themselves as to whether they are prepared to accept the risk of research for financial gain. Other critics have suggested that there should be no remuneration for participation, and that voluntary involvement should take place on an altruistic basis only.

What is clear is that coercion should be avoided, as this may erode the autonomy of the individual subject. It would be considered unethical, for example, to make the parole of prisoners or access to expensive treatments conditional on participation in a research trial.

- *Information*: Guidelines indicate that the subject should be informed, *inter alia*, of what is involved in taking part, why the research is being done, what the risks might be to the subject, and what the consequences of those risks might be. There would appear to be a far greater ethical requirement that the researcher adopt a 'full disclosure' approach to providing information to research subjects. In addition, it may be that the subject is informed that there is a likelihood of *unforeseen* or *unexpected* consequences, due to the experimental nature of research. In practice, the reverse is often the case: in order to prevent subjective bias, *less* information may actually be provided to research subjects than would be the case if a clinician was attempting to persuade a patient of the importance of treatment compliance.

- *Competence*: This invariably a question of fact: either the patient is competent to give consent, or is incompetent. Two questions are immediately apparent. Firstly, should research participants be 'super-competent'? The uncertainty attached to experimentation, together with the high level of information provision that is morally required may mean that the 'average' participant is unlikely to fully comprehend and retain the information given, and use it rationally to come to a decision. Critics of this position point out that this automatically introduces bias into the research, as the majority of a population would be excluded from participation. Secondly, does this mean that incompetent patients (e.g. unconscious intensive therapy unit (ITU) patients) should not participate in research? Can it ever be in the 'best interests' of patients to be included in a research trial without giving their consent? If this is the case, then it has been argued that there will never be any progress made in the treatment of certain diseases or disease processes (e.g. Alzheimer's, cerebral haemorrhage, sepsis syndrome) occurring in the 'incompetent' patient population, who arguably often have the most to gain from innovative therapies.

## (b) Beneficence

Two criteria are commonly accepted as ensuring beneficence in research. Firstly, the study should be scientifically valid, such that both the aims of the research are worthwhile, and the methodology is rigorous enough to provide the information sought. Poor methodology may expose subjects unnecessarily to risk, without benefiting society as a result, and may expose society to risk itself, in future.

Secondly, as stated in principle 5 of the Declaration of Helsinki:

'In medical research on human subjects, considerations related to the well-being of the human subject should take precedence over the interests of science and society.'

Scientific validity (and, by extension, moral legitimacy) improves if research trials are:

- Multicentred, which increases subject numbers, and reduces geographical bias, but may expose greater numbers to risk and introduce inconsistency in data measurement.
- Prospective, which eliminates the bias and inadequacies associated with retrospective data analysis, but necessitates experimentation involving other subjects.

- Randomised, which reduces selection bias, but means that some patients in therapeutic research will not actually be receiving the new treatment, and therefore may not be receiving any benefits from participation.
- Double-blinded, which reduces observer bias, but means that both the treatment administrator and recipient are unsure as to whether the best medical therapy is being provided.
- Placebo-controlled, which reduces subject bias, but means that the patient might not be receiving any treatment at all (and is therefore to all intents and purposes participating in non-therapeutic research that cannot be in his best interests).
- Stoppable, such that if there clearly is a difference between treatments, the trial can be stopped in order either to prevent further damage to people, or to place all patients on the more beneficial treatment. Critics have suggested that the statistical evidence for early cessation must be very rigorous indeed, to prevent inappropriate statistical interpretation of 'obvious' differences.
- Sufficiently powered, such that the number of research subjects needed to validate statistical significance is calculated prior to commencement of the trial.

Therapeutic research (e.g. controlled clinical trials), therefore, should always be beneficent in nature, such that the researchers should be confident that the proposed treatment is better than existing therapies, or no treatment at all.

## (c) Non-maleficence

In terms of research, this is related to the principle of beneficence, in that subject welfare must be maximised by minimising the degree of foreseeable harm.

Non-maleficence is a core value of non-therapeutic research. Patients can never participate in non-therapeutic research, because it is never directly in their best interests. Only volunteers, therefore, may participate. The participation of healthy volunteers demands that general principles are followed, including, for instance, the maxim that the volunteer must give their consent.

Subjects should ideally be exposed to less than minimal risk, but a universally acceptable definition of 'minimal risk' has remained elusive because the phrase can incorporate a range of consequences, prevalences and subjective discomfort. Minimal risk, for example, might describe a more commonly occurring but only mildly unpleasant side-effect, such as headache or muscle stiffness, or it may be used to describe very unlikely but very serious consequences, such as death or permanent, severe disability.

Nevertheless, the risk attached to an experimental procedure should be balanced against its possible benefits. The GMC (2002) state that:

'in non-therapeutic research, you must keep the foreseeable risks to participants as low as possible. In addition the potential benefits from the development of treatments and furthering of knowledge must far outweigh any such risks'

Other authorities (including the Medical Research Council (MRC) and the Law Commission) have added that non-therapeutic research which involves greater than minimal risk may be carried out if the disease is sufficiently common or severe, if there is no other means of obtaining the knowledge (e.g. through laboratory or animal experiments) and if the subject consents to participation, having accepted the increased risk.

## Confidentiality

Research necessarily involves the collection and retention of sensitive information about research subjects, and every effort should be made to maintain the confidentiality of these records. Prospective studies usually present few problems, inasmuch as confidential records can be formed from the time of enrolment, with the proviso that the confidentiality of the data will be maintained, and invariably anonymised. Retrospective studies are more problematic, in that consent may be unobtainable for the disclosure of necessary medical records.

The requirement for confidentiality extends to the reporting of research, such that patients should not be identifiable.

Sections 30–42 of the GMC guidelines (*Research: the role and responsibilities of doctors*) are concerned with confidentiality. In general:

'Patients and people who volunteer to participate in research are entitled to expect that doctors will respect their privacy and autonomy. Where data is needed for research, epidemiology or public health surveillance you should:

- seek consent to the disclosure of any information wherever that is practicable;
- anonymise data where unidentifiable data will serve the purpose;
- keep disclosures to the minimum necessary;

- keep up to date with, and abide by, the requirements of statute and common law, including the Data Protection Act, 1998 and orders made under the Health and Social Care Act, 2001.'

## Fraud

Fraudulence can occur at any stage of research, from the false recording of results to the deceptive reporting of research, and is suspected of being more wide spread than has been previously accepted. Fraudulent research can place lives at risk by informing doctors about their practice. In addition, it often takes time for the medical profession to actually realise that an excess of harm is occurring to patients because a piece of research has been fraudulent.

There are numerous reasons for fraud, which include the publication-based system of career advancement, the pursuit of kudos, notoriety or financial gain, and 'conflicts of interest' (e.g. not declaring drug-company sponsorship).

An interesting long running lawsuit concerning academic freedom and conflicts of interest has recently been settled in Canada, and has implications for international research. Nancy Olivieri, an internationally respected professor of haematology, won her case against Apotex Inc., the producers of an experimental drug Deferiprone, an oral iron chelator developed for use in beat-thalassaemia major. Her research, sponsored by Apotex Inc. along with the MRC of Canada, found that Deferiprone was less effective than originally supposed. When Olivieri wanted to disclose the ill effects, the company threatened to take legal action to enforce a confidentiality cause in a research contract that she had signed. Furthermore, the hospital at which Dr. Olivieri worked (The Hospital for Sick Children in Toronto) did not support her against Apotex Inc. allegedly because the hospital stood to lose money if Apotex withdrew their financial support for research. Furthermore, she was demoted from her position at the hospital. All subsequent inquiries into the conduct of the various actors completely exonerated Dr. Olivieri. The consequences of this case are far reaching, but reinforce the absolute necessity for both academic freedom in research, and constant monitoring against the very real risk of a conflict of interest occurring (leading to fraudulent research – i.e. the suppression of negative results) when substantial sums of money are involved.

The Committee on Publication Ethics (COPE) formed in 1997, is an informal collection of medical journal editors intent on monitoring and exposing publication fraud. COPE have also provided clear guidelines concerning good publication practice, dealing with areas such as study design and ethical approval, conflicts of interest and plagiarism.

## LAW

Surprisingly, there has never been any statutory law governing human experimentation in the UK (animal research is regulated by the Animals (Scientific Procedures) Act, 1986).

Specific regulation exists in three areas only:

- *Medicinal products*: The Medicines Act, 1968 regulates clinical trials on patients of unlicensed medicinal products.
- *Gene therapy*: The Gene Therapy Advisory Committee (GTAC) was established in 1993, in order to consider and advise on the acceptability of proposals for gene therapy research (therapeutic and non-therapeutic) on human subjects, with reference to the scientific merits of the proposals and their potential benefits and risks. GTAC must give its approval before gene therapy research is conducted on humans.
- *Xenotransplantation*: UK Xenotransplantation Interim Regulatory Authority (UKXIRA) – which informs the government before any research involving xenotransplantation is granted a licence.

## LOCAL AND MULTICENTRE RESEARCH ETHICS COMMITTEES

Nevertheless, some degree of extra-statutory protection is provided for National Health Service (NHS) patients in the form of Local and Multicentre Research Ethics Committees (LRECs and MRECs). Guidelines concerning the rationale, constitution and implementation for LRECs were published in 1991, and for MRECs in 1997; these were superceded by the 'Governance Arrangements for NHS Research Ethics Committees (GAfRECs)' in July, 2001.

LRECs (and MRECs if more than five centres are involved) must be consulted about any research involving NHS patients, foetal material and *in vitro* fertilisation, recently dead patients, access to past or present medical records, and use or access to NHS premises. LRECs do not cover research involving healthy volunteers. Legal liability lies with the researcher, rather than the LREC; however, committee members may be held negligent if they fail to assure themselves of certain facts relating to the research (e.g. soundness of scientific reasoning and robustness of trial design), and patient harm results. As public bodies, LRECs may be subject to Judicial Review of their decisions.

LRECs are tasked with addressing a minimum of eight questions when considering research proposals (*GAfRECs*, Section 9.13):

1 *Has the scientific merit of the research been assessed adequately?* It is not the function of the LREC to determine the scientific merit of research, merely whether the scientific merit has been adequately assessed.

2 *How will the research affect the health of the research subjects?* This relates particularly to the nature of research procedures, and their risks and consequences.

3 *Are there hazards associated with the research, and are there adequate facilities to deal with any hazards?*

4 *What is the likely degree of distress or discomfort?* This particularly relates to research in children, the mentally impaired or the otherwise incompetent.

5 *Is the research supervised by an appropriately qualified person?* Senior colleagues should ideally be actively involved in the proposed research, rather than merely providing verbal support or advice.

6 *Are there any conflicts of interest?* For example, financial, political, personal or other inducements that might affect the objectivity of the proposed research.

7 *Are there appropriate procedures in place for obtaining legally valid consent?* In addition, what are the procedures for recording discussions about consent?

8 *Is a comprehensive, and readable, information sheet to be made available to participants?* This should include information about the nature and purpose, risks and consequences, of the research, reinforce the maxim that the subject may withdraw at any time, and provide contact telephone numbers and addresses for specified members of the research team.

## COMMON LAW

If there is no statutory provision concerning research, then plaintiffs must appeal to the common law if they have a complaint.

### (1) Therapeutic research

As has been noted previously, only therapeutic research may be carried out on patients, because non-therapeutic research is not in the best interests of the patient. Consent is an absolute requirement for patient participation in therapeutic research, and must be recorded in written form. A decision must therefore be made as to whether the patient is competent or incompetent to give legally valid consent to participation in the research.

## (a) Competent patients

Competent patients (according the test in *ReMB*) may consent or refuse to participate in research, or may withdraw their consent at any time, and for whatever reason. In order to consent to research, they must do so:

- Voluntarily.
- After being adequately informed, as to the nature and purpose of the treatment intended (to avoid a claim in battery), and the risks and consequences of the treatment (to defend a claim in negligence). Kennedy and Grubb suggest, quite rightly, that in addition to the above, information must be provided concerning the research itself. Regarding nature and purpose, they suggest that the patient be told that:
  - *both* treatment and research are intended;
  - refusal to participate at any time and for any reason will not affect ongoing treatment;
  - the patient may be a member of a control group;
  - the patient may be randomly allocated to a treatment group or a control group.

To these may be added:

  - that a placebo may be used;
  - the trial may stop early;
  - any conflicts of interest on the part of the researcher;
  - a confirmation of the confidential nature of any records.

Similarly, information about the risks and consequences should additionally pertain to the experimental treatment, and mention the possibility that there may be risks yet to be ascertained.

## (b) Incompetent patients

Incompetent patients may be considered for inclusion in trials provided that the research is necessary, is in their best interests (i.e. therapeutic in nature), cannot be conducted on competent patients, and is scientifically valid as determined by an LREC. This was confirmed by

Dame Elizabeth Butler-Sloss in the recent case of *JS v An NHS Trust; JA (a minor) v An NHS Trust* [2003] 11 Med Law Rev 237, in which it was held that an experimental therapy may be used in an attempt to improve the neurological status of JS and JA, who were incompetent through having contracted variant Jakob–Creutzfeld disease (vCJD).

Children may be entered into clinical trials either if they are *Gillick* competent, although probably with a higher level of understanding than that required for the purposes of non-research medical treatment, or if proxy consent is voluntarily given by a competent, informed person who has care of the child – in addition, the child must not object to the proposed therapy.

## (2) Non-therapeutic research

Non-therapeutic research is invariably conducted using healthy volunteers. Volunteers are usually competent, but may be incompetent, to give their consent to such research.

### (a) Competent volunteers

Volunteers may take part in research if they do so:

- *Voluntarily*: Financial inducements, which might otherwise amount to coercion, should only cover reasonable expenses in terms of time, expenditure or inconvenience;
- After being adequately informed, as indicated above. Kennedy and Grubb suggest that the following additional information is provided to avoid claims in negligence:
  - a medical history should be obtained prior to the procedure;
  - the doctor should obtain permission from the patient to inform the patients doctor of his participation;
  - the doctor should ascertain that the patient is not participating in any concurrent trial;
  - the doctor should provide resuscitation facilities as appropriate;
  - the doctor must ensure that the patient is prepared to inform the doctor of any change in his circumstances.

### (b) Incompetent volunteers

Despite considerable debate, it rightly remains unethical to submit children to non-therapeutic research that exposes the child to any more than a minimal risk (accepted as 1–100/million of death, 10–100/million of major complication, or 1–100/thousand of a minor complication).

Incompetent adults are unable to give their consent to participate in research, and non-therapeutic research cannot take place in their best interests. Nevertheless, such research may be considered necessary in order to improve understanding of the disease process from which they are suffering. Several authorities, including the MRC (*The Ethical Conduct of Research on the Mentally Incapacitated* (1991)) and the Law Commission (*Mental Incapacity*), have promoted the idea that non-therapeutic research should be an acceptable practice using incompetent non-patients, but that:

- the research should significantly advance the understanding of the disease;
- the research cannot be conducted on competent volunteers;
- the participants are not exposed to any more than *negligible* risk;
- there should be a system of stringent protections in place, possibly including the assent of the courts.

The Department of Constitutional affairs has recently had the opportunity to explicitly incorporate guidance about research using incompetent patients or volunteers into statutory law in the form of the draft Mental Incapacity Bill, but, at the time of writing, has chosen not to do so.

## FURTHER READING

### Books

Kennedy and Grubb (Eds). *Medical Law*, 3rd edition. Research, Chapter 14, pp. 1665–1749

Sales BD and Folkman S (Eds). *Ethics in Research With Human Participants*, American Psychological Association, Washington, 2000

Hare RM. Little human guinea-pigs. In Hare RM (Ed.). *Essays on Bioethics*, Clarendon Press, Oxford, 1996, Chapter 9

### Journals

Angell M. The Ethics of Clinical Research in the Third World. *New Engl J Med* 1997; **337**: 847–849

Biros *et al.* Informed consent in emergency research. *J Am Med Assoc* 1995; **273**: 1283–1287

Baram M. Making clinical trials safer for human subjects. *Am J Law Med* **27(2 and 3)**, 253–282

Emanuel EJ, Wendler D and Grady C. What makes clinical research ethical? *J Am Med Assoc* 2000; **283**: 2701–2711

Freedman B. Equipoise and the ethics of clinical research. *New Engl J Med* 1987; **317**: 141–145

Ferguson PR. Legal and ethical aspects of clinical trials: the views of researchers. *Med Law Rev* 2003; **11**: 48–66

Lemaire F, Blanch L, Cohen SL and Sprung C. Informed consent for research purposes in intensive care patients in Europe – Part I. An official statement of the European Society of Intensive Care Medicine. *Intens Care Med* 1997; **23**: 338–341

Peart N and Moore A. Compensation for injuries suffered by participants in commercially sponsored clinical trials in New Zealand. *Med Law Rev* 1997; **5**: 1–21

Viens AM and Savalescu J. Introduction to the Olivieri symposium. *J Med Ethic* 2004; **30**: 1–7

## Internet

Committee on Publication Ethics. http://www.publicationethics.org.uk/

Department of Health. Governance Arrangements for NHS Research Ethics Committees (GAfREC). July, 2001. http://www.doh.gov.uk/research/documents/gafrec.pdf

General Medical Council. Research: The Role and Responsibilities of Doctors. February, 2002. http://www.gmc-uk.org/standards/default.htm

Governance arrangements for NHS Research Ethics Committees (GAfREC). (2001). http://www.dh.gov.uk/assetRoot/04/05/86/09/04058609.pdf

Medical Research Council. MRC guidelines for good clinical practice in clinical trials. http://www.mrc.ac.uk/pdf-ctg.pdf

World Medical Association. Declaration of Helsinki. http://www.wma.net/e/policy/b3.htm

# 11

# Death and organ procurement

*'I will neither give a deadly drug to anybody if asked for it, nor will I make a suggestion to this effect.'*

– Hippocratic Oath

Everyone dies. Approximately 500,000 people die per year in England and Wales. In relation to surgery, perioperative mortality is less than 2% for patients classified as American Society of Anesthesiologists (ASA) grades I, II and III (i.e. no comorbidity to severe but not incapacitating systemic disease), a figure which is increased to 8–10% in ASA IV and V patients, and particularly when emergency surgery is performed. Preceding a significant proportion of deaths is a period of high-dependency or intensive care treatment, during which the patient – who was previously competent – is rendered legally incompetent, by reason of sedation, illness or unconsciousness. In addition, there are a number of ill but competent patients, undergoing higher risk surgery, who have a significant chance of dying perioperatively.

This section is concerned with the degree to which sick or incompetent patients can influence their own treatment and discusses aspects of UK law once death has occurred.

## ETHICS

The ethics of death encompass a wide range of topics, including suicide, euthanasia and organ retrieval. However, a number of issues relating to death and dying reappear in discussions about these various topics:

- sanctity of life arguments;
- autonomy, dignity and surviving interests;
- justice and justification for killing;
- the doctrine of double effect;
- physician involvement in or detachment from dying.

## Sanctity of life arguments

These have previously been discussed in the chapter on abortion (Chapter 8). Essentially, whether society considers it is absolutely wrong to cause the death of another human or whether there are occasions in which causing death is justified, there appears to be some recognition that being alive is a very desirable state of being for humans; conversely, causing death has very limited moral acceptability, if any at all. Controversies surround what is meant by 'being alive' and whether 'being alive' (i.e. in the sense that a patient with persistent vegetative state (PVS) is still alive) is as valuable as 'being a person'.

## Autonomy, dignity and surviving interests

Society appears to accept that autonomy transcends death or the appearance of death. Citizens are able to sign wills, for example, detailing the disposal of their estates after death. Furthermore, there is an intrinsic desire that our deceased bodies are not used without regard for our personal or religious beliefs. Kantian ethics support this, in that our bodies should not be used as a means to an end after death; for example, society does not, at present, recognise dead bodies as organ banks for transplantation, without the pre-mortem consent of the deceased (utilitarianism, of course, recognises the opposite: the deceased, arguably, has no surviving interest, so only good can come out of non-consensual organ retrieval).

The ethical concept of human dignity has been incorporated into the European Convention on Bioethics and Biomedicine. Interestingly, one might argue that society gives greater reverence to the concept of human dignity *after* death than it does before death. Dead bodies are treated with respect (morally and in law) and surviving interests are recognised. However, there appears to be no general acceptance of or right to, a dignified death. This may be for two reasons. Firstly, such a right is not universally applicable. For example, soldiers who lose their lives horrifically in battle or the millions who die of starvation every year, cannot be said to be accorded a dignified death. Secondly, to allow a dignified death would allow for physician-assisted suicide. This argument recognises, for example, that a terminally ill cancer patient who is in excruciating continuous pain might deserve a dignified death, but that this would require an act by a third party that brought about death; if this were to happen, there would be a paradigm shift towards the intentional killing of less sick individuals.

## Justice and justification for killing

Are there any situations or justifications for actively killing another human being or is the proscription of killing absolute? The following circumstances provide examples that make absolute vitalism hard to defend:

- *Mercy killing*: The classic example is of the lorry driver trapped in his vehicle, who is burning to death, with no means of escape. Would a friend with a gun be justified in shooting the lorry driver in order to shorten his suffering? Critics have argued that, whatever the merits of killing the lorry driver in this scenario, this is not an analogy that can be transferred to the physician-assisted death of a terminally ill patient who suffers pain.

- *Sacrifice*: Suppose five hikers became trapped in a cave with only one exit. If the first of their number became completely trapped in the exit whilst attempting to extricate himself from the cave, would the others be justified in killing and dismembering him in order to free themselves? This is a classic utilitarian example of where the greater good may be served by killing one person in order to save the lives of four others. However, this argument could also be used to advocate the far less palatable scenario in which a demented patient with a rare blood group is exsanguinated, causing his death, in order to provide life-saving blood transfusions for four other patients.

- *Altruism*: Suppose a government 'death squad' arrests 10 people and states its intention to kill all 10 people unless one volunteer agrees to be shot and killed in order to save the lives of the other nine. Alternatively, suppose a soldier volunteers to draw the enemies' fire so that his injured comrades might survive, even though this will result in his death. In these and similar circumstances, does an individual have the right to determine how his life might end? To be sure, there is no act on the part of others that results in death, but their omission either in stepping forward to the firing squad or preventing the soldier's altruism, will result in a death occurring, even if the greater good is served. Should it be acceptable, therefore, for parents to donate organs to their children, even if donation will result in the parent's death?

- *Self-defence*: If you are attacked, and the only way of saving your own life is by killing your assailant, should you do so? A famous case is that of Simon Yates, a mountaineer who cut the rope holding his fellow climber, Joe Simpson, in order to avoid the dead weight of Simpson pulling *both* climbers off the mountain (both survived, and

Simpson wrote about the episode in his book *Touching the Void*).
A self-defence argument was also used in defence of the killing of
one twin, Mary, in order to save the life of her conjoined sister,
Jodie (*ReA (Children) (Conjoined Twins: Surgical Separation)* [2001]
2 WLR 480). Self-defence is an argument more commonly used as
a defence to abortion, the foetus being seen as the assailant.

## The doctrine of double effect

The doctrine of double effect elaborates on the nature of intention in
relation to acts that result in the death of another. The doctrine is familiar
to doctors in cases where terminal pain relief is provided: does the administration of significant doses of morphine for example, cause the patient's
death through respiratory suppression or does it allow the patient to die
in relative comfort? According to the doctrine of double effect, such an
act may be morally acceptable if (and only if):

- the action is good in itself (i.e. prevention of further pain and
  suffering);
- the intention is *only* to produce the good effect (i.e. the doctor's
  intention is only to provide relief from pain and suffering and not
  to hasten the patient's death);
- the good effect is not achieved through the bad effect (i.e. the
  death of the patient is not the thing that brings relief from pain
  and suffering);
- there is adequate reason to allow the bad effect (i.e. relief from pain
  and suffering is good and death may not be such a bad outcome in
  these circumstances).

## The acts/omissions distinction

The question concerns whether the doctor who fails to institute
life-saving treatment (an omission) is as morally culpable as the doctor
who actively brings about a patient's death (an act). Some see the distinction as irrelevant, as the consequence is the same (the patient dies),
there is intention in both the omission (i.e. electing not to intervene)
and the act (i.e. killing), and it is often less than clear cut (e.g. omitting
treatment may involve the act of discontinuing ventilation or disconnect-
ing intravenous antibiotics). Nevertheless, there remains a moral
acceptance that the intention of an omission is not to actively kill someone – after all, there is the possibility that they may yet survive (this is the
position in law, where it is not so much the withdrawal of life-sustaining

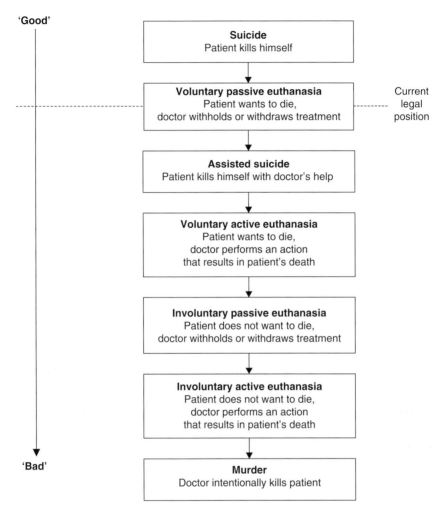

**Figure 11.1** A moral hierarchy of physician assistance in patient death.

therapy that kills the patient as the disease process from which the patient is suffering).

## Euthanasia and physician-assisted death

The terminology surrounding euthanasia is often muddled. Essentially, euthanasia represents a spectrum of activity related to death, with passive voluntary euthanasia at one end and murder at the other (Figure 11.1).

There is considerable debate in the UK at present, as to whether euthanasia should be legally recognised to the extent that it is in other jurisdictions (e.g. Holland), such that doctors may actively bring about the death of their patients, in line with the patients' choice and consent. Advocates of voluntary active euthanasia use the following arguments:

- In a civilised society, death should be a dignified process whenever practicable. This appeals to the core principle of beneficence, in that the medical profession should act in the best interests of the patient, which could include cases where the benefits of permanently alleviating pain and suffering outweighed the burden of continued existence.
- Patients should be able to determine the nature of their deaths, a position that appeals to the core principle of respect for autonomy and defers to the human rights of the patient.
- There would be some consistency reintroduced to the law. Patients are legally allowed to commit suicide if they are capable of physically doing so, including in situations where they are suffering from terminal disease. However, when that disease robs them of the physical capacity to take their own life, they also lose the legal ability of terminating their own life, as the law does not permit the aiding or abetting of a suicide.
- There should be Regulation. There is a general suspicion that doctors, through acts or omissions, covertly institute euthanasia at present. The legalisation of euthanasia, particularly with regard to improved regulation would make this unnecessary and would restore trust to the medical profession.

Opponents of euthanasia, who remain in the majority at present, cite the following arguments:

- There is no absolute right to die with dignity. Furthermore, the generally accepted 'right to life' does not confer a 'right to death'. Although not absolute in their nature, religious and moral principles accept that life is intrinsically valuable.
- Doctors are bound by the principle of non-maleficence, which is incompatible with physician-assisted suicide or euthanasia; furthermore, physician involvement is more likely than not to *erode* public trust rather than enhance it.
- Many doctors do not want to participate in euthanasia (although interestingly, these are in a slight minority).
- There is a credible slippery slope argument with euthanasia, which describes the future countenance of involuntary euthanasia or worse, and incorporates the fear that decisions could become based on questions of resource allocation. As one commentator has noted 'Once you accept killing as a solution for a single problem, you will

find tomorrow hundreds of problems for which killing can be seen as a solution'.

- Palliative care precludes the need for euthanasia. Palliative care doctors have made great strides in relieving pain and suffering, thus providing a dignified death for patients without the need for actively bringing about death.

## Organ procurement and transplantation

The legal recognition of brainstem death, coupled with medical advances both in organ-specific support of the dead donor and transplantation success, mean that cadaveric organ donation has become an increasingly viable method of securing organs for potentially life-saving transplants.

According to figures compiled by UK transplant, in the year up to April 2004, 5697 patients were awaiting organ transplant (5000 of which were awaiting kidney transplants). Organs were donated from 772 deceased donors and 457 living donors: 2397 organ transplants were carried out, 1330 of which were kidney transplants. Adult recipients wait on average 506 days for renal transplants, 164 days for heart transplants and 374 days for lung transplants (203, 73 and 1292 days, respectively, for children). It is clear from these figures that there is a significant short-fall in the supply, compared to the demand, of organs for transplantation.

Two solutions exist. Firstly, the demand for human organs could be reduced. To this end, there is considerable medical interest in both developing drugs to prevent chronic organ damage and in developing alternative technologies, such as mechanical hearts and 'portable kidneys'. Of considerable ethical interest is the discussion surrounding xenotransplantation, which involves the transplant of organs or tissues from other species into humans (e.g. pig heart valves), with opponents of this practice arguing, *inter alia*, that it is morally wrong to implant organs from other species into humans *per se*, that it is wrong to kill animals as a means to an end (i.e. merely as organ providers for humans) and that it is uncertain whether xenotransplantation might pass as yet unknown diseases onto humans.

The other solution revolves around increasing supply, which assumes greater current importance until the above technologies become more advanced. A large number of ethical issues are raised, including:

- *The national system of organ procurement:* At present, the UK has an opt-in system of organ procurement, such that individuals may elect to offer their organs for transplantation in the event of their death (by carrying a donor card or indicating their wishes in any form of advanced directive). However, only 15–20% of the UK population are registered organ donors. Furthermore, their relatives may overrule this decision after death. It has been suggested that an opt-out system would be a more effective and utilitarian way of increasing the number of organs for transplantation, by allowing the removal of any organ from any dead body, unless that person had expressly refused organ donation before death. Critics (deontologists) have argued against this, because it views people as a means to an end, is contrary to their surviving human rights and is contrary to the rule of law.

- *Payment for organs*: There is a degree of moral revulsion at this prospect, but it may have advantages. Living donors retain the choice of whether to donate their organs, and the estates of deceased donors may benefit from the sale of their organs (which may be in line with the deceased's wishes), thereby benefiting both the donor and the recipient. The concerns are that financial coercion vitiates any donor consent, that relatives may abuse the system contrary to the wishes of the deceased and that there would be considerable injustice in the rich West taking advantage of the impoverished citizens of Third World countries.

- *The definition of death*: At present in the UK, death is accepted as having occurred when there is irreversible loss of the capacity for consciousness *and* irreversible loss of the capacity to breathe, which is synonymous with brainstem death. It has been suggested that this definition could be extended to include patients with PVS, who still have the capacity to breathe but no capacity for consciousness.

- *The role of relatives/third parties*: Two issues arise. Firstly, that relatives should not be allowed to veto the deceased's request for donation; a similar veto is not recognised in other areas of law, and recognition of the rights of those legally in charge of the body after death should not be allowed to take precedence over either the patient's surviving interest in autonomy or the interests of the recipient in receiving the organ. Secondly, the regulation of non-live related donors should be relaxed, in line with the regulations for live related donors, to allow living donors who are not related to the recipient to volunteer their organs for transplant, either through altruism or for financial gain.

- *Conditional donation/receivership*: The number of donors might increase if donors were allowed to specify to whom their organs could be transplanted into. This might extend respect to the donor's autonomy, but at the expense of certain unacceptable restrictions (e.g. stating that the recipient should not be of an identified colour or religion). Alternatively, there is the question of whether organs should not be allocated to certain types of recipient, who through their behaviour are considered less deserving of transplantation (e.g. patients taking paracetamol overdoses, smokers or alcoholics), thus increasing the number of organs available for other patients.

## LAW

### Brain death

Modern technology enables doctors to maintain cardiorespiratory function (and therefore organ perfusion) despite the death of the brain. This ability has forced the medical and legal professions to reassess traditional definitions of the point at which death occurs.

Surprisingly perhaps, there is no statute that defines death in the UK. Death is considered to have occurred when there is irreversible loss of the capacity for consciousness plus irreversible loss of the capacity to breathe – that is when the brainstem dies. The condition of an intact brainstem without higher cerebral function is termed Persistent Vegetative State or PVS. That brainstem death is synonymous with 'legal death' was confirmed in *ReA* [1992] 3 Med Law Rev 303 (Fam Div) and by a majority of the House of Lords (HL) in the case of Tony Bland (*Airedale NHS Trust v Bland* [1993] 1 All ER 821 (HL)).

Tests to establish the diagnosis of brainstem death were published in the British Medical Journal (BMJ) in 1976, resulting from a Conference of Medical Royal Colleges and their faculties. The Department of Health published a similar *Code of Practice for the Diagnosis of Brain Stem Death*, in 1998 (HSC/1998/035); this is summarised below:

*Preconditions to testing:*

- there should be no doubt that the patient's condition is due to irremediable brain damage of known aetiology;
- the patient is deeply unconscious, though not due to cerebral depressant drugs, hypothermia or potentially reversible circulatory, metabolic or endocrine disturbances;
- the patient must be attached to a ventilator because spontaneous ventilation has been inadequate or has ceased altogether.

*Tests performed:*

- all brainstem reflexes are absent;
- a ventilator disconnection test confirms no spontaneous respiratory effort by the patient.

Ideally, two sets of tests should be performed several hours apart, by a different doctor on each occasion, one of which should be a consultant, both of which should have specialist knowledge in the field of brainstem death testing (e.g. intensivist, neurologist), both of which should have been qualified for more than 5 years and neither of which should be a member of a transplant team.

## Withdrawal of life-sustaining treatments

Two circumstances generally arise that require consideration of whether to withdraw or withhold life-sustaining treatment:

- there is a request by the patient;
- further treatment is considered futile or not in the best interests of the patient.

In the first instance, patients are usually competent to make the decision, are suffering from incurable and disabling conditions and seek what may be termed a 'dignified' death. In the second, the decision rests with the courts or with doctors themselves as to whether to continue treating an incompetent patient, when it is 'certain' that the patient will die from his/her current condition.

## (a) Competent patients

In English law, it is clear that a competent, informed adult patient, acting voluntarily, can refuse contemporaneous medical treatment, for any (or no) reason, rational or irrational, even if refusal results in the patient's death and even if the patient is not terminally ill. This does not apply to competent minors (*ReW (a minor)(medical treatment)* [1992] 4 All ER 627, *ReL (medical treatment: Gillick competency)* [1998] 2 FLR 810).

These legal principles were reinforced very publicly in the recent case of Ms B (*B v An NHS Trust* [2002] EWHC 429 (Fam)), a tetraplegic who refused continued artificial ventilation and followed the judgements passed in a number of other cases (*ReT (adult)(refusal of medical treatment)* [1992] 4 All ER 649, *Airedale NHS Trust v Bland* [1993] 1 All ER 821 (HL), and *St Georges Healthcare NHS Trust v S* [1998] 3 All ER 673 (CA)).

However, as was made clear in *Bland* (and *B v An NHS Trust* [2002] EWHC 429 (Fam)), in refusing life-sustaining treatment 'there is no question of the patient having committed suicide nor therefore of the doctor having aided or abetted him in doing so' (and therefore committing a criminal offence under Section 2(1) of the Suicide Act, 1961 – punishable by up to 14 years in jail).

Can a patient demand treatment beyond that which a doctor is obliged to give? Not if doctors consider that the treatment is futile (*ReJ (a minor)(wardship: medical treatment)* [1992] 4 All ER 614 (CA)) and probably not if refusal to treat was based on rational and responsible consideration of resource implications. It is also quite clear that doctors, at present, may neither accede to competent patients' requests to provide the means with which patients may kill themselves ('physician-assisted suicide') (which is in contravention of Section 2(1) of the Suicide Act, 1961) nor perform 'mercy killing' (i.e. involuntary euthanasia).

The human rights aspects of assisted suicide were examined in the recent case of Dianne Pretty, a competent woman severely physically disabled by motor neurone disease, who sought the Court's guarantee that her husband would not be prosecuted under the Suicide Act, 1961, if he helped her commit suicide. In considering her application, the HL (and the European Court in Strasbourg) rejected her claim that Article 2 (Right to Life) conferred a right to die, that Article 3 (Prohibition of torture) demanded that the government end her suffering and that Article 8 (Right to Respect for Private and Family Life) conferred a right to choose the manner of her death.

Doctors are not obliged to participate in decisions about withdrawing therapy if they conscientiously object. However, they are obliged to 'ensure, without delay, that arrangements have been made for another suitably qualified colleague to take over their role, so that the patient's care does not suffer' (General Medical Council (GMC), *Withholding and withdrawing life-prolonging treatments*).

The government has recently introduced the Patient (Assisted Dying) Bill. The bill seeks to legalise voluntary euthanasia by enabling doctors to assist patients to die who are 'suffering unbearably as a result of a terminal or a serious and progressive physical illness'. The bill states the circumstances in which such an action could be taken and provides a schedule to be signed by a patient which would authorise the doctor to end the patient's life. However, there remains considerable opposition to the passage of the bill at present.

## (b) Incompetent patients

Incompetent patients, by definition, lack the capacity for legal self-determination and therefore cannot provide a legally valid refusal of treatment. Nevertheless, decisions still have to be made as to whether treatment should be continued or withdrawn on the basis that its continuation will not improve the patient's condition or prevent further deterioration. It is important to note the gravity of these decisions, the consequences of which could result in the death of the patient.

Who should make the decision? In *ReF (mental patient: sterilisation)* [1990] 2 AC 1, the HL vested proxy decision-making for incompetent adult patients in doctors, although they suggested certain instances where court involvement would be desirable (including 'more serious' decisions). Patient's relatives are not able to refuse treatment on the patient's behalf and are not able to provide 'substituted judgements' as to what the patient might have wanted if they were competent (*Bland*), although it remains important to take relatives' views into account (*ReG (PVS)* [1995] 2 FCR 46 (Fam Div), *NHS Trust A v M; NHS Trust B v H* [2001] 2 WLR 942, GMC and British Medical Association, BMA guidelines).

Doctors have a duty to act in the best interests of incompetent patients. For dying patients, the best interests of the patient are served by the relief of pain and suffering and the cessation of 'no purpose' (i.e. futile) treatment (*ReC (a minor)(wardship: medical treatment)* [1989] 2 All ER 782 (CA)).

Two classes of 'non-dying' incompetent patients are recognised:

- The 'living dead' (i.e. PVS patients). The leading case is *Airedale NHS Trust v Bland* [1993] 1 All ER 821 (HL), in which the HL decided, *inter alia*, that discontinuation of artificial hydration and nutrition was neither the act that caused death nor a breach of the doctors' duty of care to the patient; the HL decided that the court's assent was not needed for every case of PVS and should be limited to cases where there was disagreement amongst doctors and/or the patient's relatives. In *NHS Trust A v M; NHS Trust B v H* [2001] 2 WLR 942, Dame Elizabeth Butler-Sloss identified that the criteria and approaches taken in *Bland* were compatible with Articles 2, 3 and 8 of the European Convention on Human Rights (ECHR) as enacted by the Human Rights Act, 1998 (HRA), most notably that the lack of awareness in PVS meant that suffering could not be experienced, and therefore Article 3 could not be engaged.
- Those in whom the benefits of treatment may be outweighed by its burden (e.g. major cancer surgery for demented nonagenarians). The index cases in England concerned severely disabled infants: *ReB (a minor)(wardship: medical treatment)* [1981] 1 WLR 1421 (CA) and *ReJ (a minor)(wardship: medical treatment)* [1991] Fam 33 (CA), which determined that the court, in determining whether it should authorise steps not to prolong life, should act in the best interests of the child, the best interests being dependent on consideration of

the doctors' assessment of the treatment options, the parents desire for treatment to continue and an assessment of the quality of life of the patient.

In *R v Portsmouth Hospitals NHS Trust ex parte Glass* [1999] Lloyd's Rep Med 367 (CA) the court reviewed the lawfulness of the withdrawal of life-sustaining treatment from a child without the consent of the parents. The child, now 12, was born with severe mental and physical disabilities including cerebral palsy, hydrocephalus and epilepsy. The child suffered various infections following a tonsillectomy. Clinical staff considered that the child was dying and wished to administer pain relief to alleviate his distress. The patient's mother opposed this without her consent. There were a number of violent incidents between the child's parents and the staff over this issue. The child was discharged from hospital and treated by their general practitioner (GP). The trust suggested that the child should be treated in another hospital. His parents applied for a judicial review of the trust's conduct regarding the treatment, seeking declarations regarding both the lawfulness of the treatment and the withdrawal of life-saving treatment against the wishes of the parents. The court emphasised the role of the family court in these circumstances, the importance of considering the best interests of the child and the limits of deference to medical opinion that should be shown by the courts in other such decisions.

*Glass* confirmed for minors the legal principles applicable to adult cases after the decision in *ReR (adult: medical treatment)* [1996] 31 BMLR 127 (Fam Div). This case emphasised three important points:

- 'global' orders to withhold treatment are inappropriate – instead, withholding therapy should be limited to specific treatments (e.g. no cardiopulmonary resuscitation (CPR), not starting antibiotics if their use is indicated);
- treatments may be withheld if they are considered futile, in line with professional guidelines;
- determination of quality of life and best interests appear to be restricted to doctors (with the court's opinion, if sought) and not to carers.

## Anticipatory decisions ('advance directives'/'living wills')

The above law relates to contemporaneous decisions about life-sustaining therapy. However, a third possibility exists – that of the competent patient who anticipates future incompetence and declines life-sustaining therapy (*Note*: 'Birth plans' also fall into this category). The law concerning advance directives has developed in an attempt to recognise the interest that individuals have in maintaining a continued right of self-determination.

Subsequent to *ReT (adult: refusal of medical treatment)* [1992] 9 BMLR 46 (CA) and *ReC (adult: refusal of medical treatment)* [1994] 1 All ER 819 (Fam Div), anticipatory refusals of treatment by patients are held to be legally valid if:

- a refusal of treatment is clearly established (e.g. the patient refuses blood transfusion even if it is clinically indicated);
- the patient is competent at the time of the decision;
- the patient is adequately informed at the time of the decision;
- the patient makes the decision voluntarily;
- the decision is intended to apply in the circumstances which subsequently arise (e.g. CPR should be attempted if the patient is involved in a road traffic accident when still competent, but not if the same patient requires ventilation on the intensive care unit as a consequence of future motor neurone disease).

The validity of advance directives was confirmed in the recent case of *ReAK (Adult patient) (Medical treatment: consent)* [2001] 1 FLR 129. This case concerned a 19-year old who had suffered from motor neurone disease for 2 years. In October 1999, as a fully competent adult aged 19, he informed his nursing team (in the presence of his mother) that he wished to make an advanced statement concerning his future treatment. Should he develop a chest infection, he instructed that he would like the nursing team to treat it. However, if his heart should stop he instructed that he should not be treated. In July 2000, he was informed of the impending loss of his ability to communicate. A few days later he informed his carers, with an eyelid movement, that he wished his ventilation to be stopped if he could no longer communicate. His doctor spoke to him and explained to him what would happen if his ventilator was switched off. The doctor also informed him that he would be able to administer a sedative drug to allow him to die without suffering, but that the drug itself would not shorten his life in anyway. The patient confirmed his decision on several occasions in the presence of witnesses. This decision was recorded by his carer. The care team were satisfied that this reflected his true wishes and that he was unaffected by the effect of any drug treatment. The health authority applied to the High Court for a declaration that this approach was lawful and consistent with the patient's wish to discontinue support and after 2 weeks treatment he lost the ability to communicate. The court held, following the established principles of previous case law, that an adult patient of full capacity had the right to refuse treatment, and that doctors are not entitled to carry on treatment if they are aware of this decision. To this extent, an advanced indication of the patient's wishes is effective, but great care must be taken to ensure that the advance declaration truly reflects the patient's wishes in the given circumstances. Such a case is clearly distinct from cases where a patient is in PVS where no advance decision has been stated.

In *Re AK*, Mr Justice Hughes held that an advance refusal had the same legal authority as a contemporaneous refusal. The judge outlined the criteria required in law in order for an advance refusal of treatment to be valid:

1 Doctors must be satisfied that the patient is of full capacity.
2 They must carefully examine the voluntariness of the refusal: care must be taken to investigate the circumstances in which the refusal was given, namely that the refusal was fully informed by the expected consequences.
3 Care must be taken to examine how long ago the refusal was given and whether it still represents the wishes of the patient.
4 For the refusal to be valid, it must have specifically envisaged the situation that has arisen.

The judge emphasised that there could be no active steps to encourage or act to end life, and that life can end only via the omission of continued treatment. Although the HRA had not yet come into force, he considered that this approach was compliant with the requirements of the ECHR to protect life, avoid inhuman and degrading treatment and respect privacy. He also noted that the High Court was the appropriate venue for a declaration to be made as to the lawfulness of action on an advance directive if a conflict arose.

The Draft Mental Incapacity Bill includes provisions for the statutory regulation of advance decision-making (Clauses 23–25) (Figure 11.2).

Clause 23 of the Mental Incapacity Bill asserts the lawfulness of advanced refusals of treatment by competent individuals, allows the refusal to be worded broadly and provides for withdrawal of the refusal by patients if they are competent to do so.

Clause 24 describes the circumstances under which advanced decisions would be regarded as valid and applicable, with particular emphasis placed on situations that invalidate advanced refusals of treatment. Notably, an advance decision is not applicable to life-sustaining treatment unless the patient specified that their decision was to apply to such treatment.

Clause 25 describes the effect of advanced directives and discusses liability either for withholding/withdrawing treatment or for carrying

23  **Advanced decisions to refuse treatment: general**
    (1)  In this section and Sections 24 and 25 'advanced decision' means a decision made by
         a person ('P'), after he has reached 18 and when he has the capacity to do so, that if;
         (a)  at a later time and in such circumstances as he may specify, a specified treatment
              is to be carried out or continued by a person providing health care for him,
         (b)  at that time he lacks capacity to consent to the carrying out or continuation of
              the treatment, the specified treatment is not to be carried out or continued.
    (2)  For the purposes of Subsection (1)(a), a decision may be regarded as specifying a
         treatment or circumstances even though it is expressed in broad terms or non-
         scientific language.
    (3)  An advanced decision may be withdrawn or altered by P at any time when he has
         capacity to do so.

24  **Validity and applicability of advanced decisions**
    (1)  The lawfulness or otherwise of carrying out or continuing a treatment in P's case is
         not affected by P's advanced decision unless the decision is at the material time:
         (a)  valid,
         (b)  applicable to the treatment.
    (2)  An advanced decision is not valid if P:
         (a)  withdrawn the decision at a time when he had capacity to do so,
         (b)  has, under a lasting power of attorney created after the advance decision was
              made, conferred authority on the done (or, if more than one, any of them) to
              give or refuse consent to the treatment to which the advance decision relates,
         (c)  has done anything else clearly inconsistent with the advance decision
              remaining his fixed decision.
    (3)  An advanced decision is not applicable to the treatment in question if at the
         material time P has capacity to give or refuse consent to it.
    (4)  An advanced decision is not applicable to the treatment in question if:
         (a)  the treatment is not the specified treatment in the advanced decision,
         (b)  any circumstances specified in the advanced decision are absent,
         (c)  circumstances exist which were not anticipated by P at the time of the advanced
              decision and which would have affected his decision had he anticipated them.
    (5)  An advanced decision is not applicable to life-sustaining treatment unless P
         specified that his decision was to apply to such treatment.
    (6)  The existence of any lasting power of attorney other than one of a description
         mentioned in Subsection (2)(b) does not prevent the advanced decision from
         being regarded as valid and applicable.

25  **Effect of advanced decisions**
    (1)  Subject to Subsection (2), if P has made an advanced decision which is:
         (a)  valid,
         (b)  applicable to the treatment,
              the decision has effect as if he had made it and had the capacity to make it, at
              the time when the question arises whether the treatment should be carried out
              or continued.
    (2)  A person does not incur liability for carrying out or continuing the treatment if, at
         the time:
         (a)  he does not know,
         (b)  he has no reasonable grounds for believing
              that an advanced decision exists and is valid and applicable to the treatment.
    (3)  A person who withholds or withdraws a treatment from P in the belief that a valid
         advanced decision is applicable to the treatment, is not liable for the consequences
         of doing so if his belief is reasonable.
    (4)  The court may make a declaration as to whether a valid advanced decision that is
         applicable to the treatment exists.
    (5)  Nothing in apparent advanced decision stops a person:
         (a)  providing life-sustaining treatment,
         (b)  doing any act reasonably believed to be necessary to prevent a serious
              deterioration in P's condition, while a ruling as respects any relevant issue is
              sought from the court.

**Figure 11.2** Clauses relating to advanced decisions in the draft Mental
Incapacity Bill.

out/continuing treatment. The bill is explicit in stating that nothing in an apparent advance decision stops a person from providing either life-sustaining treatment or performing any act that is reasonably believed to be necessary to prevent a serious deterioration of the incompetent person's condition, while a ruling on any relevant issue is sought from the court.

The new bill does not impose a requirement that the advance decision has to be in writing. Criminal liability only attaches to a breach of the advance decision. Presumably, other cases will be brought under common law, with civil liability in battery or according to human rights legislation.

## 'Do not resuscitate' orders

Again, no statutory law exists. The guidelines that inform clinical practice in the UK are those provided by the BMA, Royal College of Nursing and the UK Resuscitation Council joint statement of 2002. This may be summarised as follows:

### Principles

- support for patients and people close to them, and effective, sensitive communication are essential;
- decisions must be based on the individual patient's circumstances and reviewed regularly;
- information about CPR and the chances of a successful outcome needs to be realistic.

### In emergencies

- If no advance decision has been made or is known, CPR should be attempted unless:
  - the patient has refused CPR;
  - the patient is clearly in the terminal phase of illness;
  - the burdens of the treatment outweigh the benefits.

### Advance decision-making

- competent patients should be involved in discussions about attempting CPR unless they indicate that they do not want to be;

- where patients lack competence to participate, people close to them can be helpful in reflecting their views.

## Legal issues

- patient's rights under the HRA must be taken into account in decision-making;
- neither patients nor relatives can demand treatment which the health care team judges to be inappropriate, but all efforts will be made to accommodate wishes and preferences;
- in England, Wales and Northern Ireland, relatives and people close to the patient are not entitled in law to take health care decisions for the patient;
- in Scotland, adults may appoint a health care proxy to give consent to medical treatment;
- health professionals need to be aware of the law in relation to decision-making for children and young people.

Figure 11.3 provides a simplified algorithm for decision-making concerning 'do not resuscitate' orders.

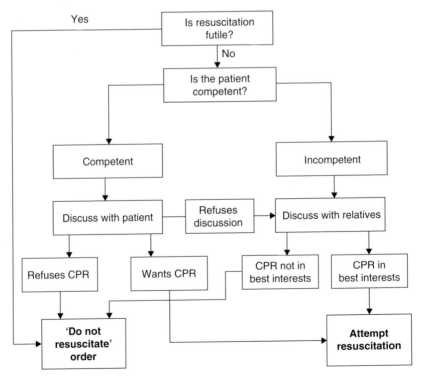

**Figure 11.3** 'Do not resuscitate' algorithm.

## Postmortems

Postmortems involve the dissection of dead bodies in order to determine the cause of death. The current hospital postmortem rate is 8%, a figure that the National Confidential Enquiry into Perioperative Death (NCEPOD) describes as 'unacceptably low'. Postmortems may be performed:

- When directed or requested by the Coroner (Sections 19–21 Coroners Act, 1988) if the Coroner has reasonable cause to suspect that a person has died a sudden death of which the cause is unknown or a violent and unnatural death, and it is his/her opinion that a postmortem may prove an inquest to be necessary (or that a postmortem is necessary after deciding to hold an inquest).
- With the authority of someone 'lawfully in possession of the body', under Section 2(2) of the Human Tissue Act, 1961 (HTA) (usually, an executor or next of kin (or their designates) or a Coroner or a hospital management committee before the body is claimed by a greater authority).

Subsequent to the Bristol Royal Infirmary enquiry, the BMA have advised that it is ethically desirable to seek relatives' informed consent before a decision is made to retain organs and tissue from the deceased for the purposes of medical education and research (see below).

## Organ donation by the deceased

Development of the concept of brainstem death permits recovery of materials for transplantation from the bodies of dead persons, even though their hearts continue to beat through artificial means and their organs remain transfused and viable for transplantation.

The functional distinction between tissues and organs is that the former tend to be donated primarily by live donors, whereas acquisition of organs is primarily from cadaveric sources. Cadaveric organ donation is regulated by the HTA. Recovery of cadaveric organs for transplantation depends in law on both the application of the legal criteria for death (i.e. brainstem death testing) and appropriate consents being given.

Donation (for therapeutic, educational or research purposes) is authorised either by patient request prior to death (provided the request was not withdrawn) or by a person lawfully in possession of the body after life is extinct, subject to the consent of the Coroner, if he is involved. Requests by the deceased are in effect anticipatory decisions (see above). Those lawfully in possession of the body may authorise donation provided they believe that the deceased had not previously objected and that a surviving spouse or other relatives do not object, 'having made such reasonable enquiry as may be practicable'.

## Deceased donors

Dead bodies have long been governed by the 'no property' rule of the common law, such that one person cannot own another as a piece of property. Nevertheless, the law requires that someone is recognised as being legally in possession of a body after death (for the purposes of burial, postmortem etc.). It is usually the executors of a deceased person's estate that have a right to lawful possession of the body. However, Section 1(7) of the HTA provides that when a body is in a hospital or nursing home, power to authorise removal of a body part for the purposes of the act may be given by a designated managerial person of that institution.

A donor who wishes to express a request that the person lawfully in possession of their body (or parts of it) be allowed to authorise the use of tissues for transplantation following death may do so by two mechanisms.

- The most common is by providing consent in writing. No specified form has been established in law. Written consent for postmortem organ donation need not be witnessed and no confirmation of capacity is required. If the donor lacked capacity or if capacity is at issue, the person who is lawfully in possession of the body may still authorise removal of body parts under Section 2(1) of the HTA, unless there is a reason to believe that the deceased objected to this use (Section 1(2)(a)). If the deceased lacked capacity and objected to donation, the person in possession ought not to override any purported objection.
- Consent to donation can also be given orally, in the presence of two or more witnesses during the donor's last illness. The last illness is a matter of medical evidence and relates to both the cause of death and the pathology of the disease. An oral statement given by someone who dies from a cause unrelated to their final illness is not sufficient for the purposes of Section 1(1) of the HTA. However, evidence of consent may support the position of the person in possession of the body under Section 1(2) regarding the validity of donation. By analogy, witnesses attest to the validity of the signature on a will and not to the competence or the intent of the will. Nevertheless, witnesses are obliged to recognise the nature of the donor's consent. Witnesses to an oral consent can also be

beneficiaries of that consent. The HTA does not impose any age limits on who can be a witness, although child witnesses are likely to have doubt cast on their capacity to be a witness.

The HTA does not specify a minimum age for the donor who wants to offer their organs. However, Section 8(1) of the Family Law Reform Act, 1969 (FLRA) provides for effective consent to medical treatment by minors aged 17 or 18. A request for donation is not 'treatment' under the FLRA, but it may provide for an analogy authorising posthumous donation. The oral statement of a person of 16 years of age or less, may only serve as support to any consent given by the person in possession of the body under Section 1(2) of the HTA (usually the parents in this instance). However, there is some doubt as to whether written donation on the part of a minor would be effective under Section 1(1) and would turn on whether the minor was competent to make that decision.

Donation by a competent adult does not compel the person in subsequent possession of the body to make it available for harvest of organs and tissues. It is clear that Section 1(1) of the HTA only describes a donation as a 'request', with the final authority transferred to the person in possession of the body. The person in possession of the body may decline the request for whatever reason. Surviving spouses and relatives of the deceased person may also object to organ harvest.

Common law respects the dignity of corpses by creating the criminal offences of causing indignity to a dead body (*Foster v Dodd* [1866] LR1 QB) and infringing public decency by improper handling of corpses (*R v Gibson* [1991] 1 All ER 439). Section 1(3) of the HTA appears to give some form of qualified defence to these offences. Section 1(1) allows for the donation of an entire body or any part of it. Section 1(4), however, limits the authorisation to obtain material such that 'no removal, except of eyes or parts of eyes, shall be effected except by a registered medical practitioner, who must has satisfied himself by personal examination of the body that life is extinct.' Acquiring material from a dead body other than as allowed by the HTA would risk prosecution. Section 1(4A) was added by the Corneal Tissue Act, 1986, and provides that no removal of an eye or part of an eye shall be exercised except by a registered medical practitioner who has personally examined that life is extinct or another person employed by a health authority and acting under the instruction of a registered medical practitioner.

## Living donors

Under Section 2(1) of the Human Organ Transplants Act, 1991 (HOTA), a person is not guilty of an offence if (s)he transplants an organ from another living person, provided the donor is genetically related to the recipient. Section 2(2) identifies 'genetically related' as including natural parents and children, whole or half-blooded brothers and sisters and children of these.

The legislation was accompanied by The Human Organ Transplants (Unrelated Persons) Regulations 1989, which provided for donation between non-blood relative donors and recipients (e.g. partners, husband and wife), as long as approval had been granted by the Unrelated Live Transplant Regulatory Authority (ULTRA).

## Payment

Section 1 of the HOTA criminalises the making or receiving of payments for the supply of organs from living or dead donors or any associated practice (e.g. negotiation, initiation or advertising). However, the distinction between organs and tissues is significant, as the prohibitions and punishments apply only to organs. Payments for tissues which are replaceable naturally, such as blood or bone marrow, are not illegal. Contractual relationships between donor, intermediary or recipient are likely to be considered void if they are contrary to public policy regarding the supply of tissues, in an attempt to prevent commercial dealings in body parts. Nevertheless, Section 1(3) of the HOTA permits payment for the costs and expenses involved in organ donation. Subsection (a) allows for reimbursement of costs associated with removal, transport and storage that will be recoverable by those in possession of the body if incurred by them.

## Supply of information

Section 3(1) of the HOTA empowers the Secretary of State to make regulations requiring specific persons to supply information to a particular authority concerning transplants from living or dead donors. Failure to comply or the provision of misleading information is a criminal offence created by this act. The Human Organ Transplants (Supply of Information) Regulations 1990 govern this supply of information.

## The Human Tissue Bill

The existing legislation of tissue and organ removal and retention for research purposes, especially in children has proven problematic as exemplified in both the Royal Liverpool (Alder Hey) Children's inquiry of 2001 (which enquired into the removal, retention and disposal of human tissue and organs following Coroner and hospital postmortem examinations and the extent to which the HTA had been complied with) and the Bristol Royal Infirmary Inquiry Interim Report of 2001 (which investigated the retention of organs after paediatric cardiac surgery). The Government is attempting to address this issue with the Human Tissue Bill. In addition to these inquires, a census by the Chief Medical Officer for England and the conclusions of the *Isaacs* Report (2003) (following the unauthorised removal and retention of Mr Isaacs brain for research purposes after his untimely death in 1987), showed that storage and use of organs and tissue from both adults and children without proper consent has been widespread in the past. It also became clear that the current law in this area was not comprehensive, nor as clear and consistent as it might be.

The purpose of the Human Tissue Bill is to provide a consistent legislative framework relating to whole body donation and the taking, storage and use of human organs and tissue. Consent will become the fundamental principle governing the lawful storage and use of human bodies, body parts, organs and tissue, and the removal of material from the bodies of deceased persons. The bill will set up a regulatory authority that is intended to rationalise existing regulation of activities like transplantation and anatomical examination and will introduce regulation of other activities like *postmortem* examinations and the storage of human material for education, training and research. It is intended to achieve a balance between the rights and expectations of individuals and families, and broader considerations, such as the importance of research, education, training, pathology and public health surveillance to the population as a whole.

In his advice to the government (*The Removal, Retention and Use of Human Organs and Tissue from Postmortem Examination* (2001)), the Chief Medical Officer recommended that there should be a fundamental and broad revision of the law on human organs and tissues taken from adults or children, either during surgery or after death.

The bill will repeal and replace the HTA, the Anatomy Act 1984 and the Human Organ Transplants Act 1989, as they relate to England and Wales.

The bill proposes three main areas of legislation.

- *Part 1 – Consent*: There will be a requirement to obtain appropriate consent to carry out activities regulated under the bill, namely the storage and use of whole bodies, the removal, storage and use of human material (organs, tissues and cells) from the bodies of deceased persons and the storage and use of material from living people. It defines 'appropriate consent' (and who may give it), and provides for a 'nominated representative' who may make decisions about regulated activities after a person's death. It will be a criminal offence to carry out regulated activities without appropriate consent, making it unlawful to use bodies or human material, once donated, for purposes other than those described in the bill. Part 1 of the bill also sets out what should happen to 'existing holdings' of human material obtained before the consent provisions take effect. Part I exempts coroners from these requirements and additionally allows the storage and use of human material, obtained from living persons, for limited purposes without consent. Part 1 does not apply to the removal (as opposed to the storage and use) of human material from living persons, and the current law will continue to apply.

- *Part 2 – Regulation of activities involving human tissue*: The bill proposes the formation of a Human Tissue Authority (HTA), whose remit covers the removal, storage, use and disposal of human material and relevant licensing procedures and responsibilities. Part 2 also brings the regulation of all living donor transplants under the aegis of the HTA and prohibits commercial dealing in human material.
- *Part 3 – Supplementary issues and general provisions*: Clause 44 makes it clear that it is lawful for hospital authorities to take the minimum steps to preserve the organs of deceased persons whilst appropriate consent to transplantation is sought. Clause 46 makes it an offence, with specified exceptions, for a person to have human material with a view to analyse its deoxyribonucleic acid (DNA) without consent (which has implications for research and criminal justice).

## FURTHER READING

### Books

Glover J. *Causing Death and Saving Lives*. Penguin, London, 1990

Kennedy and Grubb (Eds). The end(ing) of life: competent and incompetent patients. In: *Medical Law,* 3rd edition. Chapters 16 and 17, pp. 1905–2190

Kennedy and Grubb (Eds). Death and dead bodies. In: *Medical Law*, 3rd edition. Chapter 18, pp. 2191–2233

Kennedy and Grubb (Eds). Donation and transplant of human tissues and fluids (from 'the dead donor'). In: *Medical Law*, 3rd edition. Chapter 15, pp. 1832–1848

Pallis C and Harley DH. *ABC of Brainstem Death*, 2nd edition. BMJ Publishing, London, 1996

Steinbock B and Norcross A (Eds). *Killing and Letting Die*, 2nd edition. Fordham University Press, New York, 1994

Zucker MB and Zucker HD. *Medical Futility*. Cambridge University Press, Cambridge, 1997

## Journals

Allmark P. Death with dignity. *J Med Ethic* 2002; **28**: 255–257

Fox M and McHale J. Xenotransplantation: the ethical and legal ramifications. *Med Law Rev* 1998; **6**: 42–61

Harris J. The survival lottery. *Philosophy* 1975; **50**: 81–87

Harris J. Human beings, persons and conjoined twins: an ethical analysis of the judgment in *ReA*. *Med Law Rev* 2001; **9**: 221–236

Harris J. Consent and end of life decisions. *J Med Ethic* 2003; **29**: 10–15

Harris J. Organ procurement: dead interests, living needs. *J Med Ethic* 2003; **29**: 130–134

Kerridge IH, Saul P, Lowe M, McPhee J and Williams D. Death, dying and donation: organ transplantation and the diagnosis of death. *J Med Ethic* 2002; **28**: 89–94

Nesbit W. Is killing no worse than letting die? *J Appl Phil* 1995; **12**: 101–105

Onwuteaka-Philipsen BD, van der Heide A, Koper D. *et al.* Euthanasia and other end-of-life decisions in the Netherlands in 1990, 1995, and 2001. *Lancet* 2003; **362**: 395–399

Park GR. Death and its diagnosis by doctors. *Br J Anaesth* 2004; **92**: 625–628

Price D. From Cosmos and Damian to Van Velzen: The human tissue saga continues. *Med Law Rev* 2003; **11**: 1–47

Rachels J. Active and passive euthanasia. *New Engl J Med* 1975; **292**: 78–80

Rachels J. Killing and starving to death. *Philosophy* 1979; **54**: 159–171

Sheldon S and Wilkinson S. 'On the sharpest horns of a dilemma': *ReA (Conjoined twins)*. *Med Law Rev* 2001; **9**: 201–207

What is a good death? *Br Med J Theme Issue* 26th July, 2003

White SM, Baldwin TJ and Miss B. *Anaesthesia* 2002; **57**: 818–819

Williams G. The principle of double effect and terminal sedation. *Med Law Rev* 2001; **9**: 41–53

## Internet

British Medical Association. Decisions Relating to Cardiopulmonary Resuscitation Decisions Relating to Cardiopulmonary Resuscitation. A Joint Statement from the British Medical Association, the Resuscitation Council (UK) and the Royal College of Nursing, 2002. http://www.bma.org.uk/ap.nsf/650f3eec0dfb990fca25692100069854/0a4960b756b615f180256b41003e012f/$FILE/Cardiopulmonary.pdf

British Medical Association. Physician Assisted Suicide – the Law. http://www.bma.org.uk/ap.nsf/Content/Physician+assisted+suicide%3A+The+law

British Medical Association. Withholding and Withdrawing Life-Prolonging Medical Treatment. Guidance for Decision-Making. http://www.bmjpg.com/withwith/contents.htm

British Medical Association. Interim BMA Guidelines on Retention of Human Tissue at Post-Mortem Examination for the Purposes of Medical Education and Research, 2000. http://www.bma.org.uk/ap.nsf/Content/Retention+of+human+tissue+at+post-mortem

Chief Medical Officer. The Isaacs Report. http://www.publications.doh.gov.uk/cmo/
    isaacsreport/
Department of Health. Code of Practice for the Diagnosis of Brain Stem Death, 1998.
    (HSC/1998/035). http://www.dh.gov.uk/assetRoot/04/03/54/62/04035462.pdf
Draft Mental Incapacity Bill, 2003. http://www.dca.gov.uk/menincap/meninc.pdf
General Medical Council. Cardiopulmonary Resuscitation, 1999.
    http://www.gmc-uk.org/standards/cpr.htm
General Medical Council. Withholding and Withdrawing Life-Prolonging treatments.
    Good Practice in Decision-Making, 2002. http://www.gmc-uk.org/standards/
    whwd.htm
National Confidential Enquiry into Perioperative Deaths (NCEPOD).
    http://www.ncepod.org.uk/reports.htm
Patient (Assisted Dying) Bill. http://www.parliament.the-stationery-office.co.uk/
    pa/ld200203/ldbills/037/2003037.pdf
Resuscitation Council (UK). The Legal Status of those who Attempt Resuscitation, 2000.
    http://www.resus.org.uk/pages/legal.htm
The BBC. Religion and Ethics. Euthanasia.
    http://www.bbc.co.uk/religion/ethics/sanctity_life/deathindex.shtml
The Bristol Royal Infirmary Inquiry. Interim Report: Removal and Retention of Human
    Material. http://www.bristol-inquiry.org.uk/interim_report/index.htm
The Human Tissue Bill. http://www.parliament.the-stationery-
    office.co.uk/pa/cm200304/cmbills/009/04009.i-v.html
The Royal Liverpool Children's Inquiry. http://www.rlcinquiry.org.uk/download/

## Legal cases

*Airedale National Health Service Trust v Bland* [1993] AC 789 (HL)
*B v An NHS Trust* [2002] EWHC 429 (Fam)
*NHS Trust A v M; NHS Trust B v H* [2001] 2 WLR 942
*Pretty v Director of Public Prosecutions and Secretary of State for the Home Department*
    [2001] UKHL 61
*ReA* [1992] 3 Med Law Rev 303 (Fam Div)
*ReAK (Adult patient)(Medical treatment: consent)* [2001] 1 FLR 129
*ReJ (a minor)(wardship: medical treatment)* [1992] 4 All ER 614 (CA)
*ReC (a minor)(wardship: medical treatment)* [1989] 2 All ER 782 (CA)
*ReR (adult: medical treatment)* [1996] 31 BMLR 127 (Fam Div)

# 12
# Professional regulation

*'To hold him, who has taught me this art, as equal to my parents, and to live my life in partnership with him, and if he is in need of money to give him a share of mine, and to regard his offspring as equal to my brothers in male lineage, and to teach them this art if they desire to learn it without fee and covenant; to give a share of precepts and oral instruction and all the other learning to my sons and to the sons of him who has instructed me, and to pupils who have signed the covenant and who have taken an oath according to the medical law, but to no one else.'*

– Hippocratic Oath

Can anyone call themselves a doctor? No, according to Section 49(1) of the Medical Act, 1983:

> 'any person who wilfully and falsely pretends to be or takes or uses the name or title of physician, doctor of medicine, licentiate in medicine and surgery, bachelor of medicine, surgeon, general practitioner or apothecary, or any name, title, addition or description implying that he is registered under any provision of this act … shall be liable on summary conviction to a fine.'

What is it, therefore, to be able to call oneself a doctor, and why does the state recognise doctors as a specialist group whose professional name requires legal protection? This chapter deals with these questions, in addition to highlighting the quasi-legal regulation of the profession in the UK, and recent, significant changes to that regulation.

## THE PROFESSION OF MEDICINE

A number of occupations claim to be professions, for example, the medical profession, the legal profession and the civil service. A profession may be defined as a specialised work function in society, performed by professionals committed to public welfare. More specifically, 'profession' refers to areas that require extensive study and mastery of specialised knowledge (as opposed to 'occupation', which refers generally to the nature of a person's employment). Sociologists have defined professionalism as 'organised exclusivity along guild lines', such that people external to the profession are not party to specialist knowledge, which is guarded jealously by the profession.

In addition, a professional body acts as a central administrator for members of the profession, and may have a number of functions, including: the administration of self-regulation and disciplinary procedures, the setting of professional standards, licensing procedures and the examination and certification of specialist knowledge. In the case of the medical profession, the General Medical Council (GMC) acts as the overarching legal regulator of licensed medical practice, whereas the British Medical Association (BMA) and the Royal Colleges act as quasi-legal guarantors of particular professional skills.

Medicine, as a profession, often finds itself in conflict with the state, and with citizens of the state. Doctors have legal and ethical duties of care to patients, and the trusting nature of the doctor–patient relationship, means that doctors may influence the life of the patient in ways that the state may not. The importance of trust between patients and doctors should not be underestimated; medicine is the most trusted of the occupations, but an erosion of trust makes medicine more amenable to state control (as has occurred, to an extent, in the wake of the Bristol paediatric heart enquiry, and recent scandals over retained organs) and less likely to inspire confidence in patients.

The state affords the medical profession its licence to practise. In addition, the state recognises the value of (and continuing search for) the specialist knowledge possessed by the medical profession, to the extent that organs of the state (e.g. the courts) will defer to the medical profession in matters pertaining to medicine. In return, the medical profession agrees to provide medical treatment for citizens of the state. However, professional ethics ally the medical profession more with the citizen than the state. Positive public image, a monopoly of expertise and the threat of sanctions (e.g. refusal to work, or co-operate with new policies) mean that, in a democracy, doctors can form powerful groups, and can influence the politics of the state. This is often manifest as lobbying to protect self-interest, but also means that doctors are able to resist political dogma that might be detrimental to the health of patients.

In addition, it is worthwhile to point out that doctors are themselves citizens of the state, and that this can influence their relationships with both the state and other citizens. Similarly, some doctors have a 'dual role' as members of the establishment (e.g. Government health advisers, police surgeons, public health doctors, and doctors in the armed forces), which inevitably leads to conflicts of interest between themselves, their profession, citizens and the state.

## THE GENERAL MEDICAL COUNCIL AND PROFESSIONAL CONDUCT

Established in 1858, the GMC acts as a state-sanctioned self-regulator of the medical profession, with the stated purpose of 'protecting, promoting and maintaining the health and safety of the community by ensuring proper standards in the practice of medicine'. To this end, the GMC licenses medical practice in the UK.

Until July 2003, the GMC had 104 members, twenty-five of which were lay members who represented the public. Lay and medical members take part in all stages of complaints procedures. However, government, medical and public dissatisfaction with the efficacy and accountability of the GMC in the wake of both the Bristol heart surgery enquiry and the case of Dr Harold Shipman, forced the GMC into reviewing its complaints and regulatory procedures, or face the possibility of the medical profession losing its self-regulation in favour of a state-administered form of supervision.

In December, 2002, the Privy Council agreed to proposals for reform of the GMC. The proposals covered three areas:

- *Constitutional reform*: In order to 'act more quickly and effectively', the new Council (established 1 July, 2003) consists of 35 members, 19 elected medical members (with clean criminal records, proposed by at least 10 doctors, and voted for in a nationwide ballot), two appointed medical members (nominated by the Academy of Medical Royal Colleges, and the Council of Heads of Medical Schools) and 14 lay members, appointed by the Privy Council. A member's term of office is 4 years, and they may continue in office for up to 8 years. The President is elected for a maximum of 6 years.
- *Reform of the fitness to practise procedures*: See below.
- *Revalidation*: See below.

Statutory legal powers are bestowed on the GMC by the Medical Act, 1983 (subsequently amended by The Medical Act, 1983 (Amendment) Order 2002 (SI 2002 No. 3135)), which allows the GMC to:

- regulate doctors in all branches of medicine, including hospital medicine and general practice, whether in the National Health Service (NHS) or in private practice;
- investigate any complaint received, whether it is from a member of the public, from another doctor or from a public authority (e.g. health authorities, NHS trusts or the police).

Part II of the Medical Act, 1983 concerns medical education and registration in the UK and part V professional conduct and fitness to practise. Inclusion on the Medical Register (Section 2) confers certain privileges upon the doctor, such that medicine may not be practised by a person not on the medical register (Section 49) (a criminal offence).

## COMPLAINTS

Prior to 2004, complaints to the GMC were initially assessed by a screener, a doctor. Before rejecting a complaint at this stage, the concurrence of a lay member was required. Complaints were categorised into one of three streams:

- *Conduct*: A Preliminary Proceedings Committee (PPC) initially reviewed all the evidence, with a degree of lay input. The PPC would then proceed in one of four manners: they could refer the case for a public hearing before the Professional Conduct Committee (PCC), send the doctor a letter of advice or warning, refer the case for investigation of the doctor's health or decide no further action should be taken.
- *Performance or health*: Separate performance and health procedures were followed, and hearings were held in private. If the investigation found a serious problem of performance or health, a mutually co-operative solution may have been sought. If the doctor did not agree to the GMC's suggestions, or if the public were believed to be at immediate risk, the case was referred to a PCC.

The GMC were empowered to reprimand doctors if they found evidence of:

- 'serious professional misconduct' – that is, conduct measured against the GMC's 'Good Medical Practice' standards, which leads to consideration of whether a doctor should be allowed to continue to practise medicine without restriction. According to Lord Mackay in *Doughty v General Dental Council* [1987] 3 All ER 843 (PC), a two stage test should inform the definition of 'serious professional misconduct' (as no statutory definition exists), namely that the doctors conduct should fall short, by act or omission, of the standard of conduct among doctors, and that if so, the failing should be 'serious';
- 'seriously deficient' performance – that is, the doctor is repeatedly failing to meet expected professional standards;

- criminal conviction by a British court;
- serious illness affecting a doctor's ability to practise.

Reprimands ranged from a warning letter to restriction/removal of the doctor's licence to practise. The PCC's decision to impose conditions on registration, suspend or strike off a doctor took effect about 28 days after it was announced. Doctors could appeal to the Judicial Committee of the Privy Council against the decision to suspend registration or impose conditions, within 28 days of imposition.

However, the GMC was heavily criticised for its management of patient complaints in a number of cases which highlighted deficiencies in complaints procedures and provided timely guidance for future cases (*R v GMC, ex parte Toth* [2000] Lloyd's Rep Med 368 (QBD), *Krippendorf v GMC* [2001] Lloyds Rep Med 9 (PC), *Selvanathan v GMC* [2001] Lloyds Rep Med 1 (PC). In addition, The Human Rights Act, 1998, particularly Articles 6(1), 6(2) and 7, was viewed as having the potential to alter future professional regulation. Critics had noted that NHS and GMC tribunals were not held in public, did not take place within a reasonable time, and were not heard by an independent or impartial tribunal established by law. Article 6(1) requires that there be a public hearing, but it can provide for the exclusion of the press and public under certain circumstances, such as public order, national security or protection of the privacy of certain individuals.

In turn, as part of its general reform, the GMC reviewed its complaints procedure, in order to streamline events such that they were dealt with as 'promptly as is consistent with achieving fairness'.

Therefore, from 2004, a new single complaints process was introduced. In future, all complaints will go through the same process, such that a doctor's fitness to practise will be considered overall, rather than being labelled early on as a problem of health, or of performance or of conduct. The same impositions and sanctions will now apply to every case, as appropriate. No council members will sit on the panels that decide the case against a doctor, and all panellists will be appropriately assessed for suitability.

Initially, the Registrar now assesses whether a complaint or information engages the fitness to practise procedures. The Registrar may refer convictions resulting in prison sentences direct for hearing. The need for further action is the responsibility of the Investigation Committee who are expected to delegate many of its investigation functions to Case Examiners.

Cases concerning impaired fitness to practise will in future be heard by Fitness to Practise Panels, who replace the existing PCC, Health

Committee and Committee on Professional Performance. For cases not referred to the Fitness to Practise Panel, there is a new power to issue warnings after the investigation stage.

Formal guidance now exists on the interpretation of the rules and on the procedures to be followed. Hearings are to be held in public, unless decided otherwise.

It should be remembered that patients may also complain via the NHS complaints system; 125,000 complaints are received by the NHS each year. Two-thirds of complaints made about the NHS relate to hospital care, with 46% of cases concerned with medical treatment and 39% about rudeness or the poor attitudes of staff. Four stages are recognised:

- local resolution – that is, the patient deals with the hospital concerned;
- local employment of a conciliation service;
- independent review, by a panel consisting of: a lay chair (nominated from a list of people held by the Department of Health), a convener, and a third person (either from the local Primary Care Trust or from the Department of Health list);
- involvement of the health service commissioner (who is independent of the NHS and the Government).

However, in 1999 a national evaluation of the NHS complaints procedure revealed a lack of public confidence in this system, with a general feeling that complaints procedures were lengthy, insufficiently independent and inconsistent in their decisions. The Department of Health therefore decided that a new complaints system should be formed, with a second stage run by the independent Healthcare Commission.

From 2004, complainants will be able to approach any member of staff for immediate resolution of simple complaints, and will be able to appeal to the Healthcare Commission if they fail to receive satisfaction. The time limit for making a complaint is extended from 6 months to 1 year. A further set of measures has been introduced to improve liaison between services. NHS organisations and primary care practitioners now have a duty to work together when investigating complaints that concern multiple services so that complainants receive a single, comprehensive response.

## REVALIDATION

The third core component of the recent GMC reforms concerns revalidation. With the aim of ensuring 'that doctors are up to date and fit to practise medicine throughout their careers', no doctor will be allowed by law to practise medicine without a valid licence from 1 January 2005. Doctors will be able to remain on the medical Register without a licence to practise, but will not be able to exercise any of the privileges of registration.

To maintain a licence to practise, doctors must take part in revalidation, normally once every 5 years, to show them that they have been practising medicine in line with the standards set out in the 'Good Medical Practice' standards published by the GMC. Revalidation is a two-way process: the doctor must provide evidence, and the GMC must confirm the acceptability of this evidence.

Three possible outcomes may occur through the revalidation process:

- *Revalidation*: The doctor's licence to practise will remain valid.
- *Insufficient information*: The GMC will seek further evidence from the doctor, before reconsidering the doctor's case.
- *Inadequate information*: The GMC is not persuaded by the information the doctor has provided, including any additional information that was asked for, that they should be revalidated.

The GMC will be able to withdraw a licence, but only if:

- it is no longer wanted by the doctor (e.g. retirement);
- the doctor does not pay the appropriate fee;
- the doctor fails revalidation, or does not take part in the revalidation process when asked;
- a Fitness to Practise Panel directs that the doctor's registration should be suspended or erased.

Doctors will have the right of appeal against any decision to withdraw, or refuse to restore, their licence to practise.

## SICK DOCTORS

Doctors are ordinary people, and are therefore subject to the same illnesses and stresses as the rest of the population. However, a significant body of research has been reported showing that doctors are more prone to certain illnesses than are other members of society.

Gautam, writing in the American Medical Association's recently published *Handbook of Physician Health*, notes a number of factors that may increase the risk of depression and anxiety, for example, amongst doctors including biological factors (gender, age, family history, lack of sleep, poor eating habits, poor level of fitness and physical illness), psychological factors (perfectionism, sense of responsibility, need for control, self-doubt) and environmental factors (patients' demands, professional, institutional and legal scrutiny, occupational hazards, clinical governance, personal life and work-life balance). To these may be added medical seniority (consultants feeling greater responsibility than juniors), lack of support (from colleagues, institutions or professional bodies), the ethos of perioperative medicine (i.e. to *improve* the patient's condition, through surgery), work-related exposure to death and critical illness and possibly the personality types attracted to a career in perioperative medicine.

The Association of Anaesthetists of Great Britain and Ireland (AAGBI) have previously noted that as many as 30% of anaesthetists feel stressed a lot of the time, and that stress-related behaviour, including alcoholism, drug abuse and suicide, is particularly prevalent amongst anaesthetists, compared to other medical specialities. Whereas the prevalence of addiction to alcohol and other drugs in the general population is estimated to be approximately 10%, a 1998 study of junior doctors in Newcastle-upon-Tyne reported that 60% exceeded the recommended safe limits for alcohol consumption, 36% of males (20% of females) used cannabis and 13% of males (10% of females) used other illicit drugs. The BMA estimates that 1 : 15 doctors in the UK may suffer from some form of dependence on alcohol and/or other drugs, which equates to approximately 13,000 doctors, and suggests 400–500 new cases per year.

The fitness to practise of all of these doctors will be impaired. It is important, therefore, that assistance is provided to the doctor *before* any harm accrues, either to patients or the doctor themselves. However, such individuals present a problem: doctors are notoriously reluctant to access professional help when coping with psychological stress or illness, fearing such an admission indicates personal weakness, and goes against the perceived 'cope until you croak' culture of medicine. It is crucial that, in the absence of self-referral, colleagues recognise the signs of stress or depression in a doctor, and take steps to help that individual, possibly involving the doctor's general practitioner, the departmental director, or assistance via any number of professional bodies (e.g. the AAGBI's Sick Doctor Scheme, the Sick Doctor's Trust, the BMA's Doctors for Doctors scheme, or the National Counselling Service for Sick Doctors). This is not a proposition that many doctors feel comfortable with, but bearing in mind professional commitment to clinical governance, the ramifications of legal intervention and the fact that doctors respond well to treatment, particularly for anxiety and depression, it is one that should be seriously considered.

## WHISTLE BLOWING

Doctors (or other health professionals), it would seem, are morally obliged to inform the appropriate authorities if they suspect that a medical colleague is not fit to practise. Indeed, the GMC explicitly support this notion in *Good Medical Practice*:

> '26. You must protect patients from risk of harm posed by other doctor's, or other health care professional's, conduct, performance or health, including problems arising from alcohol or other substance abuse. The safety of patients must come first at all times. Where there are serious concerns about a colleague's performance, health or conduct, it is essential that steps are taken without delay to investigate the concerns to establish whether they are well-founded, and to protect patients.
>
> 27. If you have grounds to believe that a doctor or other healthcare professional may be putting patients at risk, you must give an honest explanation of your concerns to an appropriate person from the employing authority, such as the medical director, nursing director or chief executive, or the director of public health, or an officer of your local medical committee, following any procedures set by the employer. If there are no appropriate local systems, or local systems cannot resolve the problem, and you remain concerned about the safety of patients, you should inform the relevant regulatory body. If you are not sure what to do, discuss your concerns with an impartial colleague or contact your defence body, a professional organisation or the GMC for advice.
>
> 28. If you have management responsibilities you should ensure that mechanisms are in place through which colleagues can raise concerns about risks to patients.'

However, informing the authorities of these concerns leaves the individual open to allegations of 'whistleblowing', which can have marked personal implications for the whistleblower themselves (ostracism, loss of livelihood or reputation). Nevertheless, the law supports the individual who intends to divulge his concerns:

- *Common law*: When disclosure is in the public interest, when the public interest in disclosure of information imparted in confidence outweighs the public interest in non-disclosure, particularly when there is a danger to the health or safety of others (*Woolgar v Chief Constable of Sussex Police* [1999] 3 All ER 604 (CA)).
- *Statute*:
  – Section 15, Health Service Commissioners Act, 1993, Section 24(6) Health Act, 1999 – which allow public disclosure of concerns by bodies such as the Health Commission.

– Public Interest Disclosure Act, 1998: This act encourages people to raise concerns about malpractice in the workplace, and helps to ensure that organisations respond by addressing the message rather than the messenger, resist the temptation to cover up serious malpractice, and promote the public interest through protecting whistleblowers from dismissal and victimisation.

The act applies to people at work raising genuine concerns about crime, civil offences (including negligence, breach of contract, breach of administrative law), miscarriage of justice, danger to health and safety or the environment and the cover up of any of these. It applies whether or not the information is confidential. A disclosure in good faith to a manager or the employer will be protected if the whistleblower has a reasonable suspicion that the malpractice has occurred, is occurring or is likely to occur. Where a third party is responsible for the matter this same test applies to disclosures made to it. The act protects disclosures made in good faith to prescribed bodies, including the Health Commission, where the whistleblower reasonably believes that the information and any allegation in it are substantially true.

Where the whistleblower is victimised in breach of the act he can bring a claim to an employment tribunal for compensation, although the act only provides limited protection against dismissal or suffering a detriment (e.g. being overlooked for promotion at work).

Gagging clauses in employment contracts and severance agreements are void if they conflict with the act's protection.

## PRIVATE PRACTICE

Roughly 10–15% of the population of the UK is insured or elects to pay for private health care. A number of reasons may underlie this: private health insurance is offered by the patient's employers, patients are not prepared to join waiting lists for treatment, patients would like to be treated by consultants, or patients prefer the improved facilities at private hospitals.

A minority of doctors in the UK work exclusively in private healthcare. For most, private healthcare is undertaken outside of regular work for the NHS. Until recently, full time NHS employees were entitled to participate in significant amounts of private practice in return for foregoing 10% of their NHS salary. In the future, with the new contract, it would appear that doctors will have to offer extra clinical sessions to the NHS instead.

Private practice issues are mentioned briefly throughout the rest of this book. What concerns us here are questions of probity, particularly in relation to the conduct of private medicine. It is of primary importance to note that generally, the tenets of medical practice are as applicable to the private sector as they are to medicine practised in the NHS. However, the law relating to doctor–patient relationships in the context of private medicine additionally relates to contract law (i.e. the law relating to promises, guarantees and agreements that are legally enforceable).

The International Code of Medical Ethics, adopted by the Third General Assembly of the World Medical Association in 1949, explicitly states *inter alia*:

- A doctor must always maintain the highest standards of professional conduct.
- *A doctor must practise his profession uninfluenced by motives of profit.*
- The following practices are deemed unethical:
  - any self-advertisement except, such as expressly authorised by the national code of medical ethics;
  - receiving any money in connection with services rendered to a patient other than a proper professional fee, even with the knowledge of the patient.
- A doctor ought to behave to his colleagues as he would have them behave to him.
- A doctor must not entice patients from his colleagues.

Further guidance is to be found in *Good Medical Practice* (GMC):

'Probity
*Providing information about your services*:
48. If you publish information about the services you provide, the information must be factual and verifiable. It must be published in a way that conforms with the law and with the guidance issued by the Advertising Standards Authority.
49. The information you publish must not make unjustifiable claims about the quality of your services. It must not, in any way, offer guarantees of cures, nor exploit patients' vulnerability or lack of medical knowledge.

*Financial and commercial dealings*:
53. You must be honest and open in any financial arrangements with patients. In particular:
  - you should provide information about fee and charges before obtaining patients' consent to treatment, wherever possible;
  - you must not exploit patients' vulnerability or lack of medical knowledge when making charges for treatment or services;
  - you must not put pressure on patients to accept private treatment;

– if you charge fee, you must tell patients if any part of the fee goes to another doctor.
54. You must be honest in financial and commercial dealings with employers, insurers and other organisations or individuals.

*Financial interests in hospitals, nursing homes and other medical organisations:*
57. If you have a financial or commercial interest in an organisation to which you plan to refer a patient for treatment or investigation, you must tell the patient about your interest. When treating NHS patients you must also tell the health care purchaser.'

Complaints about doctors acting in a private capacity may be referred to the GMC, as detailed above, the referral being made by the patient or by the private hospital.

Concerns about substandard care and conditions, and the handling of complaints in the private sector were addressed in 1999 by the government, who recommended these issues should be dealt by the National Care Standards Commission (NCSC). Since 1 April 2004, the NCSC has been subsumed into the Commission for Healthcare Audit and Inspection (CHAI – the Healthcare Commission).

## FURTHER READING

### Books

Gautam M. Depression and anxiety. In: Goldman LS, Myers M, and Dickstein LJ (Eds). *Handbook of Physician Health.* American Medical Association, Chicago, 2000, pp. 80–93
Green M and McConnochie K. *Clinical Negligence and Complaints: a Clinician's Guide.* RSM Press, London, 2002
Helliwell P. Sick or inadequate colleagues. In: Scott WE, Vickers MD, and Draper H (Eds). *Ethical Issues in Anaesthesia.* Butterworth Heinemann, Oxford, 1994, Chapter 12, pp. 153–162
Kennedy and Grubb (Eds). Regulation of health professionals, discipline and complaints. In: *Medical Law,* 3rd edition. Chapter 3, pp. 145–268

### Journals

Burrows J. Telling tales and saving lives: whistleblowing-the role of professional colleagues in protecting patients from dangerous doctors. *Med Law Rev* 2001; **9**: 110–129
Chambers R and Maxwell R. Helping sick doctors. *Br Med J* 1996; **312**: 722–723
Commentary. General Medical Council: complaints procedures. *Med Law Rev* 2001; **9**: 57–63

Commentary. The General Medical Council and seriously deficient conduct. *Med Law Rev* 2001; **9**: 63–67

Commentary. The General Medical Council and serious professional misconduct. *Med Law Rev* 2001; **9**: 67–70

Commentary. Fitness to practice procedures: reforming the General Medical Council. *Med Law Rev* 2001; **9**: 70–72

Wienberg A and Creed F. Stress and psychiatric disorder in healthcare professionals and hospital staff. *Lancet* 2000; **355**: 533–537

## Internet

The General Medical Council. http://www.gmc-uk.org

The General Medical Council. Duties of a Doctor. http://www.gmc-uk.org/standards/doad.htm

The General Medical Council. Good Medical Practice, May 2001. http://www.gmc-uk.org/standards/default.htm

The General Medical Practice. Helping Doctors Who are Ill: The GMC's Health Procedures. http://www.gmc-uk.org/global_sections/sitemap_frameset.htm

The Medical Act 1983, as amended by The Medical Act 1983 (Amendment) Order, 2002. http://www.gmc-uk.org/about/legislation/medical_act.htm

Department of Health. Complaints – Listening … Acting … Improving, 1996. http://www.doh.gov.uk/complaints/finalguidance.PDF

The General Medical Practice. Fitness to Practice. Proposed New Rules and Guidance. http://www.gmc-uk.org/probdocs/consult_2003/rules_consultation.doc

The General Medical Council. Licence to Practice and Revalidation for Doctors, April 2003. http://www.gmc-uk.org/revalidation/index.htm

Association of Anaesthetists of Great Britain and Ireland. Stress in Anaesthetists, 1997 http://www.aagbi.org/pdf/28doc.pdf

The Public Interest Disclosure Act 1998. http://www.legislation.hmso.gov.uk/acts/acts1998/19980023.htm

Public Concern at Work. http://www.pcaw.co.uk/

## Legal cases

*Darnell v UK* [1991] 69 DR 306

*Roylance v General Medical Council* [1999] Lloyd's Rep Med 139 (PC)

*McCandless v General Medical Council* [1995] 30 BMLR 53 (PC)

# 13

# Resource allocation

It is sometimes said that the entire gross domestic product (GDP) of the UK, or indeed any country, would be insufficient to pay for the healthcare of its citizens. In fact, only about 7% of the GDP of the UK is spent on healthcare, roughly equivalent to £1000 per person per annum (these figures are marginally lower than the equivalent values in Germany and France, and approximately half the equivalent values of the US).

With limited funds and increasing demand for ever more expensive therapies, it is inevitable that a degree of resource rationing occurs, rationing that undoubtedly leads to the problems of healthcare provision. Intensive care bed and staff availability, waiting lists, 'postcode prescribing' and hospital mergers are all examples of the consequences of rationed resource allocation.

Since the inception of the National Health Service (NHS) in 1948, successive governments have faced two politically contentious problems, namely:

- how much of the GDP should be allocated to healthcare,
- how this sum of money should be most effectively allocated.

On the whole, governments have responded in a utilitarian manner, by trying to treat as many people as possible, rather than affording high quality, expensive treatment for fewer patients.

Unfortunately, there is no single theory of health economics that adequately and effectively allocates resources. This chapter reviews the two main theories of resource allocation in healthcare (needs theory and cost-effectiveness), before outlining the development of the law in relation to resource allocation in the NHS.

## ETHICS

In an ideal world, an individual who needs medical care should have that need met. If you are fit and well, you receive nothing but pay tax anyway, with the expectation that you will receive healthcare should you subsequently require it when you become ill. This is the essence of needs theory. Needs theory is an example of distributive justice, a deontological process of resource allocation (i.e. 'healthcare should be provided if needed, because that is the moral thing to do'), that is contrary to the more contemporary utilitarian perspective (i.e. 'healthcare should be provided to maximise the welfare of the greatest number of patients').

The theory of distributive justice – the distribution of scarce resources according to fairness – was developed by John Rawls (published 1972). Rawls attempted to redefine how resources should be distributed in a just society, away from utilitarianism and towards consumerism, based on rational individual (i.e. patient) choice. By using an intriguing thought experiment, Rawls suggested that, given a choice, rational individuals would choose to live in a society in which the poorest members were maximally wealthy in comparison to the poorest members of other societies.

Norman Daniels applied Rawlsian theories of justice to healthcare, suggesting that any theory of healthcare needs should serve two central purposes. Firstly, it should illuminate the sense in which society considers healthcare special, and thus treated differently from the pursuit of other social goods. This would incorporate the widely held view that there are special reasons of justice for distributing healthcare more fairly. Secondly, a theory should provide a means of distinguishing the relative importance of various aspects of healthcare, so as to place greater value on certain aspects of treatment rather than others.

The advantages of needs theory as applied to perioperative medicine are obvious (Table 13.1):

- Those who need treatment receive treatment, even if the treatment is expensive, prolonged and not guaranteed to have a good outcome (e.g. intensive care therapy, and major surgery at the extremes of age).
- A 'basic standard' of care is provided and funded for all.

However, there are also several disadvantages:

- Expensive treatment may be given to patients who are unlikely to recover, resources that could be more appropriately and effectively spent on curing the less ill.
- Similarly, small increments in the basic level of healthcare may only be bought with an enormous financial outlay.
- A measure of inefficiency may be introduced. For example, the use of new, expensive anaesthetic drugs with marginally improved

**Table 13.1** A summary of the advantages and disadvantages of needs theory and cost-effectiveness analysis, as applied to perioperative healthcare.

|  | Needs theory | Cost-effectiveness analysis |
|---|---|---|
| Advantages | • Patients who need treatment receive treatment<br>• Basic standard of care provided | • Efficient<br>• Large numbers of patients receive treatment |
| Disadvantages | • Expensive<br>• Inefficient | • Complicated calculations involved<br>• Rationing, particularly of expensive or questionably effective treatments<br>• Ageist |

side-effect profiles would be warranted, rather than the continued use of cheaper, but effective, pre-existing formulations.

In practice the NHS was set up to meet the healthcare needs of the population, regardless of the spending power of individual citizens. However, consistently insufficient funds have been made available to meet this need. Instead, a necessary calculation of cost-effectiveness is factored into all decisions about resource allocation. Cost-effectiveness analysis provides a utilitarian method of allocating resources, such that money is spent in order to maximise healthcare benefits for a given population. Examples of cost-effectiveness strategies include day-care surgery units, preventative medicine and the redistribution of clinical duties to 'allied health professionals'.

A well-known and tested cost-effectiveness approach to resource allocation is the quality-adjusted life year (QALY). 1 QALY represents the summation of various aspects of both the quality and quantity of life remaining to a patient. A cost per QALY may be calculated per treatment. The cheaper this figure, the more 'beneficial' the treatment is to society. For example, screening programs (e.g. breast cancer, at £6800 per QALY (1996)) are considered a more beneficial method of allocating resources than waiting for a disease to occur and then treating it (e.g. breast conserving surgery followed by radiation therapy, at approximately £130,000 per QALY (2003)). Similarly, total hip replacement (approximately £2000 per QALY, depending on age), which is seemingly the standard media measure of cost-effectiveness (as in 'x number of hip replacements could be bought for the amount the government intends to spend on this new project'), could be viewed as a more efficient use of resources than, for example, triple vessel coronary-artery bypass grafting in a patient with moderate angina (£6300 per QALY).

The advantages of QALYs as a measure of cost-effectiveness include:

- the maximisation of efficiency within a healthcare system;
- their relative ease and universality of calculation and application, within a rigid economic policy;
- they may be used as an indicator for the efficient prioritisation of healthcare services.

However, the posited disadvantages of QALYs are numerous (which has led to the search for other more accurate, quantifiable measures of resource allocation), and include:

- The quality of a persons life is a subjective assessment. The remaining quantity of a persons life is an uncertainty based on survival data. The summation of quality and quantity as a definitive figure on which to base healthcare economics, therefore, is potentially inaccurate and unsound.
- QALYs are essentially unjust. If a patient is old, very ill, or likely to derive minimal benefit from treatment, they are less likely to receive adequate resources.
- 'Quality' calculations are narrow in scope, and often fail to take into account, for example, some of the social aspects of a patient's life (effect on family of illness, job prospects, leisure activities, etc.).

Are there treatments that society should not fund? In terms of peri-operative care, several contentious examples may be listed about which there is uncertainty as to whether precious public resources allocated for treatment:

- *Patients at the extremes of age.* Either very expensive treatments for severely ill neonates and infants with limited life-expectancy (e.g. some cardiac surgical procedures), or treatments for the very elderly (e.g. Coronary artery bypass graft (CABG) in the over 80 age group) have been criticised as cost ineffective.
- *Lifestyle diseases.* It has been suggested that diseases occurring as a consequence of personal activities, such as smoking or excessive alcohol intake, should require either a measure of financial input from the patient or a relative reduction in resource allocation towards those patients. Critics have pointed out that the definition of 'personal responsibility' illnesses would inevitably continue to be broadened, and might in future include, for example, human

immunodeficiency virus (HIV)/sexually transmitted disease (STD) infection through sexual practices, alcohol related trauma, sports or work related injuries, and disease related to passive smoking in the spouses or children of smokers; this would effectively penalise large sections of society, which is seen as unjust in relation to the perceived fundamental right to receive free healthcare.

- Cosmetic procedures (including gender re-assignment surgery), particularly for patients without pre-existing deformity. Some health service trusts are considering restricting or stopping access to these procedures, in order to reallocate resources.

- *Fertility procedures*: The government has recently announced its intention to fund at least one cycle of in vitro fertilisation (IVF) per couple who remain childless after 3 years of trying to get pregnant. Critics have suggested that there is no 'right to fertility', and that the money would be more efficiently spent on other areas of healthcare.

- Suicide attempts that fail, but result in severe trauma, particularly those who require prolonged intensive therapy unit (ITU) therapy.

It is often suggested that patients who fall into these categories should either not receive treatment at all, or should have to pay for the treatment themselves. However, the patient may have a general need for treatment, and the benefits to the patient themselves may be incalculable. Observers have noted that this is an unacceptable extension of utilitarian thinking, that could potentially exclude an ever increasing number of patients from receiving medical attention, leaving only those with 'worthy' diseases liable to benefit from free treatment. It should be reiterated that there remains a general acceptance of the ethos of the NHS, that 'healthcare should be freely available for all at the point of access and according to need'.

In summary, a single method of fairly distributing limited resources efficiently and according to need is yet to be developed. Consequently, grievances are always likely to arise, between financially restrained healthcare providers (both nationally and locally) and individuals or groups of patients. It is often necessary for these issues to be resolved through the process of law.

## LAW

### The traditional approach

In the UK, the majority of health care is provided for by the state. The obligations of the Secretary of State for Health are founded on the principle that they have a legal duty to promote a 'comprehensive health service'.

Section 1 of the National Health Service Act, 1977 (NHSA) imposes the following duty on the Secretary of State for Health:

'to continue the promotion ... of a comprehensive health service designed to secure improvement (a) in the physical and mental health of the people of those countries, and (b) in the prevention, diagnosis and treatment of illness for that purpose to provide or secure the effective provision of services in accordance with this Act.'

This primary duty is expanded upon in Section 3(1) of the NHSA, and schedule 8 to the Act:

'It is the Secretary of State's duty to provide ... to such extent as he considers necessary ... to meet all reasonable requirements –

(a) hospital accommodation;
(b) other accommodation for the purpose of any service provided under this Act;
(c) medical, dental, nursing and ambulance services;
(d) such other facilities for care of expectant mothers and nursing mothers and young children as he considers are appropriate as part of the health service;
(e) such facilities for the prevention of illness, the care of persons suffering from illness and the after-care of persons who have suffered from illness as he considers are appropriate as part of the health service;
(f) such other services as are required for the diagnosis and treatment of illness.'

Sections 17 and 18 of the NHSA also provide for a set of specified health service functions (listed in secondary legislation) that the health authorities are obliged to provide on behalf of the Secretary of State. Examples of these include the provision of accident and emergency and ambulance services.

The extent of the duty of the Secretary of State to provide a comprehensive health service was considered in 1980 by the Court of Appeal in *R v Secretary of State for Social Services and others, ex parte Hincks* [1992] 1 BMLR 93. The case concerned plans for a new orthopaedic unit in a hospital in Birmingham, which were approved by the Secretary of State in 1971. However, in 1973 the Secretary of State postponed the plans, and subsequently they were abandoned. It was acknowledged that there was a clear need for the service, but that, at that it was not a sufficient priority in the overall scheme of local health finance at that time.

Via the process of judicial review, the claimants alleged that the Secretary of State had failed in his duty to provide a comprehensive health service in their area. Given that the Secretary of State had approved the building of the unit and had acknowledged the need for such services, the claimants argued that Section 3(1) of the NHSA obliged the Secretary of State to provide funds in order to discharge his duty. The claimants argued that Section 3(1) did not express any limitations on the duty to discharge this function. However, the Court of Appeal decided that Section 3(1) of the NHSA cannot impose an absolute duty to provide health services irrespective of national decisions made in light of economic circumstances. Lord Denning MR to qualified the Secretary of State's duty as 'to meet all reasonable requirements such as can be provided within resources available'. Lord Justice Bridge added that the issue of resource provision 'must be determined in light of Government economic policy.'

A similar approach has been taken by the Courts when considering allocation of resources for people awaiting treatment in hospital. In *R v Secretary of State, ex parte Walker* [1992] 3 BMLR 32, a Health Authority was satisfied that a premature baby boy required an operation to repair his heart. However, the operation was cancelled due to staff shortages in intensive care. The claimant alleged that her baby was denied the surgical care that he needed and sought an application for the operation to be performed. In dismissing the claimant's application Sir John Donaldson MR stated that:

> 'It was not for this court, or indeed any court, to substitute its own judgment for the judgment of those who are responsible for the allocation of resources. This court could only intervene where it was satisfied that there was a prima facie case, not only of failing to allocate resources in a way which others would think that resources should be allocated, but of a failure to allocate resources to an extent which was *Wednesbury* ... unreasonable' (i.e. unreasonable to the extent that no reasonable authority would make that decision).

In essence, the judge stated that the court has no jurisdiction to interfere with decisions to allocate resources for health care unless those decisions are made irrationally or unlawfully (see below). However, it should be noted that Mr Justice Macpherson, in the lower court in *Walker*, stated that at the date of the hearing there was no evidence of danger to the baby, but that if an emergency arose that the operation would have to be performed. In other words, a threat to life may require the decision-maker to reallocate resources in order to protect the life of the patient.

Resource decisions concerning patients whose life or health is at risk were examined by the Court of Appeal in *R v Central Birmingham Health*

*Authority, ex parte Collier* [unreported, 1988]. The case concerned a four-year-old boy with a cardiac septal defect (hole in the heart), who urgently required correctional 'open-heart' surgery. The operation was cancelled on three occasions over a period of several months, due to lack of post-operative intensive care facilities, and had still not be carried out by the time of the hearing. An order was sought from the Court of Appeal to carry out the operation, as the boy was likely to die otherwise. However, the Court of Appeal in *Collier* merely applied the legal principles from *Walker* even though there was an imminent danger to life. *Collier* considered that the Court was in no better position than the health authorities to determine the allocation of resources.

A similar approach to *Collier* was taken in *R v Sheffield Health Authority, ex parte Seale* [1995] 25 BMLR 1, where the claimant was refused IVF treatment because she was 37 years of age, 2 years above the age limit set by the health authority for this treatment. The claimant alleged that this policy was contrary to the law set out in Section 3 of the NHSA. However, the court held that the allegation was unfounded, and that an age limit was not an irrational or absurd factor when determining the clinical merits of each case (interestingly, at the time of writing, the government is set to guarantee at least one cycle of IVF treatment for all women who remain infertile after 3 years of trying to become pregnant naturally).

## THE *WEDNESBURY* TEST, THE HUMAN RIGHTS ACT, 1998, AND HEALTH CARE PROVISION

The courts do not have any particular expertise in allocating scarce health resources. When their guidance has been sought, invariably the courts have deferred to the expertise of managers, administrators and doctors. Moreover, the courts recognise that health resource allocation, as part of general social policy, is largely a political issue. However, the courts have reserved the right to review the legality and quality of decision-making by administrators, managers, doctors and politicians. Judicial review may be used to establish the legality of either the procedure by which or the grounds on which decisions relating to resource allocation were reached.

The power to review the rationality of an administrative decision was described as follows by Lord Diplock, in (*CCSU v Civil Service* [1985] AC 374, 410):

'it applies to a decision which is so outrageous in its defiance of logic or of accepted moral standards that no sensible person who had applied his mind to the question to be decided could have arrived at it. Whether a decision falls within this category is a question that judges by their training and experience should be well equipped to answer, or else there would be something badly wrong with our system.'

The function of the Administrative court, therefore, is not to substitute its own judgment on the merits of a case, but merely to review the legality and the procedure by which a decision was made.

The approach of the courts to this issue may be slightly more stringent when assessing a decision that impacts on the human rights of the subject. The context of a judicial review is important, a point emphasised by Lord Steyn in *R v Secretary of State for the Home Department, ex parte Daley* [2001] 3 All ER 433. This case reaffirmed that the court, when dealing with human rights or issues arising under judicial review, should not conduct a review on the merits of treatment. Nevertheless, greater proportionality may operate in respect of judicial review where Convention rights under the Human Rights Act, 1998 are at stake. This was explained by Lord Steyn in *ex parte Daley*, such that the intensity of review is more stringent and less deferential to the power of decision-making of the public body concerned, when deciding on an issue with reference to its human rights implications.

For example, in *R v Cambridge HA ex parte B* [1995] 2 ALL ER 129, the concept of higher order rights were alluded to by Mr Justice Laws, in a stringent review of a decision to deny experimental life saving treatment to a child (Jaymee Bowen) suffering from leukeamia.

In *R v North East Devon HA, ex parte Couglan* [1999] Lloyd's Rep Med 306, the Court of Appeal held that the Health Authority acted unfairly in closing accommodation and transferring a disabled patient to other accommodation which was in clear breach of a promise that this would be her home for life. The argument related to the claimant's rights under Article 8 of the Human Rights Act. In addition, it was argued that the Health Authority had misinterpreted its statutory obligations under the NHSA when setting its eligibility criteria form long-term care.

In *North West Lancs HA v A, D and G* [1999] 53 BMLR 148, the Court of Appeal held that a Health Authority's decision not to fund the claimants' gender re-assignment surgery was unlawful and irrational since there had been a failure to consider the claimants' true clinical condition, and the policy of not providing any such treatment unlawfully fettered the exercise of discretion by the authority.

In *R v Secretary of State for Health, ex parte Pfizer Ltd* [2000] 51 BMLR 189, it was held that a circular advising general practitioners (GPs) not to prescribe Viagra other than in exceptional circumstances was unlawful, because it unlawfully limited the clinicians' discretion to prescribe according to need.

In summary, it is increasingly apparent that the courts are unwilling to intervene, or review, decisions concerning resource allocation, where there are broad national policy decisions at stake, but more willing to review and scrutinise decisions that affect individual people and their human rights.

## FURTHER READING

### Books

Health resources and dilemmas in treatment. Mason JK and McCall Smith RA (Eds). *Law and Medical Ethics*, 6th edition. Butterworths, London, 2002

The provision of medical care. Kennedy I and Grubb A. *Medical Law*, 3rd edition. Butterworths, London, 2000. Chapter 2

Rawls J. *A Theory of Justice*, Belknap Press, Harvard, 1972.

Newdick, C. Who Should We Treat? Law, Patients and Resources in the NHS, Clarendon Press, Oxford, 1995

Rescher N. The allocation of exotic medical lifesaving therapy. In: Kuhse H and Singer P (Eds). *Bioethics – An Anthology*, Blackwell publishers, Oxford, 1999. Chapter 41, pp. 354–365

### Journals

Daniels N. Health-care needs and distributive justice. *Phil Pub Affairs* 1980; **10**: 147–176

Harris, J. Qalyfying the value of life. *J Med Ethic* 1987; **13**: 117–123

# Appendix: Important legal cases

There are a number of legal cases in the field of medical law that are important either because they establish or confirm a legal principle, or because a number of principles are discussed during their hearing. Referred to in the text, these cases listed are more fully described below.

| Case | *Airedale National Health Services (NHS) Trust v Bland* [1993] *AC 789* (HL) |
|---|---|
| Consideration | Does the withdrawal of non-futile medical treatment render doctors liable for causing an incompetent patients death? |
| Facts | Anthony (Tony) Bland, 21-year old, suffered cerebral hypoxia having received chest injuries after being crushed in the 1989 Hillsborough football stadium disaster, and entered a persistent vegetative state (PVS). In PVS, the brainstem remains alive, and the patient can breathe. However, higher brain functions are irreparably damaged, and the patient is unable to communicate, or eat or drink unaided, and has no prospect of regaining consciousness. <br><br> Three years after the disaster, Airedale NHS Trust applied for a court ruling to decide the legality of both withdrawing artificial hydration and nutrition, and omitting to provide further medical treatment except pain relief. |
| Decision | At first instance, the declaration sought was granted. An appeal was dismissed. A further appeal was unanimously dismissed by the House of Lords. |
| Ratia | <ul><li>Doctors are under no absolute obligation to prolong a patient's life.</li><li>The test to determine a doctor's duty to an incompetent patient is that of 'best interests'.</li><li>It is the doctor who applies the 'best interests' test.</li><li>Artificial hydration and nutrition (i.e. basic care) constitutes 'medical treatment', and so may be withdrawn if they are not in the patients best interests.</li><li>Withdrawal of treatment (i.e. the doctor's act) does not cause the patient's death, rather death is a result of the patient's underlying condition.</li><li>Active euthanasia, including the administration of a drug to bring about death, is unlawful.</li></ul> |

| Case | *ReAK (Adult patient)(Medical treatment: consent)* [2001] 1 FLR 129 |
| --- | --- |
| Consideration | Are advanced directives legally binding? |
| Facts | AK, a 19-year old, had suffered motor neurone disease for 2 years, and had progressed to the 'locked in' stage, in which he retained his intellectual capacity, but was rapidly losing the power to communicate. He required 24-h care and artificial nutrition and hydration. AK made an advance statement proscribing both continued ventilation if he was unable to communicate in future, and cardiopulmonary resuscitation (CPR) if his heart stopped. The health authority sought a declaration that it would be lawful for their employees to concur with AK's wishes, 2 weeks after AK lost the power to communicate. |
| Decision | The declaration was granted. |
| Ratia | • Anticipatory decisions are lawful if it is known that the patient was of sound mind and full capacity at the time the decision was made, and that, in the event of a significant time having elapsed, this still represented their true wishes. <br> • Reaffirmed *Bland, ReT.* <br> • Valid advance directives are compliant with the European Convention on Human Rights. |

| Case | *B v A NHS Trust* [2002] EWHC 429 (Fam) |
|---|---|
| Consideration | Is the contemporaneous refusal of medical treatment – even if it leads to the patient's death – recognised by law? |
| Facts | In 1999, 41-year-old Miss B suffered a cervical cord cavernoma haemorrhage. She made a good recovery initially, and returned to work after a period of recuperation. During this period, she executed a living will, proscribing life-saving treatment in the event of future permanent mental impairment or unconsciousness. In 2001, she suffered a rebleed which resulted in tetraplegia, necessitating permanent ventilation. Her doctors disregarded her advance directive because its provisions were not considered relevant to her circumstances. A month later, after surgery to decompress the haemorrhage, she asked for ventilation to be withdrawn. Her competence to decide on withdrawal was initially confirmed by two consultant psychiatrists, but subsequently rejected when both changed their opinion a day later. Following several further reassessments, the hospital accepted Miss B's legal competence in August 2001, but continued to seek independent advice about the process of treatment withdrawal until legal proceedings were issued by Miss B in January, 2002. |
| Decision | The declaration sought was granted, namely that Miss B was 'competent to make all relevant decisions about her medical treatment, including the decision whether to seek withdrawal from artificial ventilation'. |
| Ratia | • It is reaffirmed that competent, adult patients have the 'absolute right to refuse to consent to medical treatment for any reason, rational or irrational, or for no reason at all, even where that decision may lead to his or her own death'.<br>• If there is disagreement between any parties about treatment withdrawal, declaratory relief should be sought from the courts as a matter of urgency.<br>• Withdrawal of treatment should be expedited as soon as a patient expresses a competent refusal.<br>• The case reaffirms that it is not the withdrawal of treatment, is not the act which kills the patient, rather it is the disease process itself from which the patient dies.<br>• Doctors may conscientiously object to withdrawal of treatment: 'If there is no disagreement about competence but the doctors are for any reason unable to carry out the wishes of the patient, their duty is to find other doctors who will do so.' |

| Case | *Bolam v Friern Hospital Management Committee* [1957] 1 WLR 582 |
|------|------|
| Consideration | What is the standard of medical care expected of a doctor in order to defend a case of negligence? |
| Facts | Mr Bolam suffered a fractured hip after receiving electroconvulsive therapy (ECT) without having received a relaxant drug, or being correctly restrained. He contended that the hospital was vicariously liable for the negligence of the doctor who administered the ECT. |
| Decision | The jury found for the hospital. |
| Ratia | <ul><li>By professing to have a special skill, doctors are held to the standard of the reasonable person possessing that skill.</li><li>Negligence results when the doctor fails to meet the standard of the reasonably competent medical men at the time.</li><li>'Reasonable' practice is not the same as 'accepted' or 'common' practice. A doctor may not be negligent, therefore, if experimental or unusual treatments are used.</li><li>It is for the court to decide whether there is a responsible body of medical opinion that supports the defendant.</li></ul> |

| Case | *Bolitho v City and Hackney Health Authority* [1997] 4 All ER 771 (HL) |
|---|---|
| Consideration | Who decides the standard of care in cases of alleged negligence, and what is the basis for their decision? |
| Facts | A 2-year-old boy, Patrick, who suffered from croup, died subsequent to a cardiorespiratory arrest. Patrick's mother proceeded against the Health Authority. It was commonly agreed that intubation before the respiratory arrest would have prevented progression to cardiac arrest and brain damage. However, the defendants argued that due to the risks of anaesthetising and intubating a sick 2-year-old child (Patrick having twice previously recovered to a stable state), the doctor, if she had attended Patrick prior to the respiratory arrest, may still have not intubated Patrick. |
| Decisions | • At first instance, the judge accepted the doctor's assertion that she may still not have intubated Patrick, as an acceptable standard of care.<br>• The Court of Appeal dismissed an appeal by Patrick's mother.<br>• The House of Lords unanimously dismissed Patrick's mother's appeal. |
| Ratia | • Challenged *Bolam*.<br>• The responsible body of medical opinion relied upon, when deciding the standard of care, had to demonstrate that it's opinion had a logical basis: 'In particular in cases involving … the weighing of risks against benefits, the judge before accepting a body of opinion as being responsible, reasonable or respectable, will need to be satisfied that, in forming their views, the experts have directed their minds to the question of comparative risks and benefits and have reached a defensible conclusion of the matter.'<br>• 'If professional opinion is not capable of withstanding logical analysis, the judge is entitled to hold that the body of opinion is not reasonable or responsible' that is, it is for the *court* to decide qualitatively whether the standard of care is that which is supported by a responsible body of medical opinion (rather than quantitatively whether there is a responsible body of medical opinion).<br>• That is, medical practices based on habit or experience, and not updated by current medical opinion, may not be defensible, which may, in part, underlie the increasing prominence of evidence-based medicine and practice guidelines. |

| Case | *ReC (adult: refusal of medical treatment)* [1994] 1 All ER 819 (Fam Div) |
|---|---|
| Consideration | What issues does a doctor have to take into account in order to determine whether someone is competent to give their consent to medical treatment? |
| Facts | C, a 68-year-old chronic paranoid schizophrenic (and convicted murderer) detained at Broadmoor psychiatric hospital, developed gangrene of the right lower leg. His surgeon strongly suggested below-knee amputation as a curative treatment. C contested that he would rather die with two feet than live with one. C consented to local debridement and skin grafting. C's solicitor requested an undertaking from the hospital that they would not amputate in future, in view of C's repeated refusals. The hospital sought the court's guidance as to whether C was competent to refuse treatment. |
| Decision | The judge decided that C was competent to make contemporaneous refusals of treatment. |
| Ratia | • Reaffirmed a competent patient's right to refuse treatment, even if the treatment is potentially lifesaving.<br>• A three-stage test of competency was adopted to assess competence:<br>  – That the patient could *comprehend* and *retain* the necessary information.<br>  – That the patient was able to *believe* the information.<br>  – That the patient was able to *weigh* the information, balancing risks and needs, so as to arrive at a choice.<br>• That 'mental' patients should not automatically be considered incompetent to decide on their medical treatment. |

| Case | *Chester v Afshar* [2002] EWCA Civ 724 (CA) |
|---|---|
| Consideration | What is the standard of information required of doctors in order to defend an allegation of negligence? |
| Facts | Miss Chester suffered excessive motor and sensory nerve damage after elective lumbar microdiscectomy for recurrent back pain. She contested that if she had been informed of the 1–2% risk of serious nerve damage attached to the operation, she would not have consented to the operation without further opinion or reflection, so great was her fear of being 'crippled'. |
| Decisions | • At first instance, Mr Afshar had not been found negligent in terms of the surgical operation, but the court accepted that a causal link had been established between Mr Afshar's failure to inform Miss Chester of the risks, and Miss Chester sustaining nerve damage.<br>• Mr Afshar's appeal was dismissed. |
| Ratia | • Previously, courts have been reluctant to accept the arguments of claimants had they been warned of the risks beforehand they would not have undertaken treatment.<br>• However, now 'Where a doctor, in breach of duty, fails to draw a particular risk to the patient's attention and that specific risk materialises, causative responsibility will lie. It is not necessary for the patient to prove that she would have refused the operation for all time had she been given the proper advice …' that is, a patient can recover damages in negligence if (s)he can prove that *but for* the doctors breach of duty in providing specific risk information (s)he would not have consented to an operation in that instance.<br>• This potentially increases the burden on the doctor in providing preoperative risk information. |

| Case | *ReF (mental patient: sterilisation)* [1990] 2 AC 1 (HL) |
|---|---|
| Consideration | What are the circumstances under which an incompetent patient may be given medical treatment without formal consent? |
| Facts | F, a 36-year-old very mentally handicapped woman residing voluntarily at a mental hospital, had formed a sexual relationship with a male patient. The hospital sought a declaration that it would be lawful, and in F's best interests, to sterilise her, as all other forms of contraception were unsuitable, and it would be undesirable to curtail F's access to the male patient. |
| Decisions | • At first instance, the declaration was granted.<br>• An appeal by the Official Solicitor was dismissed by the Court of Appeal.<br>• The House of Lords upheld the original declaration. |
| Ratia | • Affirmed that treatment of incompetent adults is lawful.<br>• Delineated under what circumstances such treatment would be justified (i.e. necessity, in the patients best interests. Controversially, the doctor was deemed to be acting in the best interests of a patient if a responsible and competent body of relevant professional opinion supported the doctors decision – the *Bolam* test). |

| Case | *Gillick v West Norfolk and Wisbech Area Health Authority* [1986] AC 112 (HL) |
|---|---|
| Consideration | Are children below the age of consent legally entitled to make decisions about medical treatment without the involvement of their parents? |
| Facts | Mrs Victoria Gillick, a mother of four daughters under the age of 16, wrote to the Area Health Authority to seek an assurance that, until they had reached the age of 16, none of her daughters would be provided with contraception or abortion advice or treatment without her knowledge and consent. The Health Authority refused to give any assurance. Mrs Gillick sought a declaration that a Government circular that proposed that such advice may be given to girls under 16 years of age was unlawful, because she asserted that children under the age of 16 were unable to give legally valid consent. |
| Decisions | • At first instance, the declaration was not granted.<br>• The Court of Appeal overturned this decision, supporting Mrs Gillick.<br>• The House of Lords, by a majority of three to two, overturned the decision by the Court of Appeal. |
| Ratia | • A child under the age of 16 who is deemed competent (i.e. has sufficient understanding and intelligence to enable a full understanding of what is proposed) may give consent to medical treatment.<br>• The child's competence is a question of fact.<br>• If the child is deemed incompetent, proxy consent is required.<br>• Parental assent should still be sought. |

| Case | *ReMB (an adult: medical treatment)* [1997] 2 FLR 426 (CA) |
|---|---|
| Consideration | What are the criteria for deciding the competence of a patient with regards their ability to consent or refuse medical treatment? |
| Facts | MB, 23-year old, consented to Caesarian section for breech position baby at term, but refused the insertion of an intravenous line for anaesthesia, citing fear of needles. The health authority sought, and obtained, a declaration from the court that it would be lawful to perform a caesarian section without the patients consent. MB appealed that decision. The next day, she agreed to caesarian section, and delivered a healthy baby boy. *Inter alia* MB appealed on the bases that: (1) The judge was wrong to declare her incompetent. (2) That it was unlawful to impose medical treatment on a mentally competent patient. |
| Decision | The Court of Appeal found: (1) MB was competent to refuse treatment. (2) Reasonable force (including restraint) could be used on incompetent patients for whom medical treatment was in their best interests (although it was not required in this case). |
| Ratia | Lord Justice Butler-Sloss's conclusions were exceptionally clear, and currently inform decisions about a patient's capacity to consent or refuse treatment:<br><br>• 'Every person was presumed to have the capacity to consent to or to refuse medical treatment unless or until that presumption was rebutted.<br>• A competent woman who had the capacity to decide might, for religious or other reasons whether rational or irrational or for no reason at all, choose not to have medical intervention even though the consequence might be the death or serious handicap of the child or her |

*(Continued)*

own death. In that event the court did not have jurisdiction to declare medical intervention and the question of her own best interests, objectively, did not arise.

- Irrationality connoted a decision which was so outrageous in its defiance of logic or of accepted moral standards that no sensible person who had applied his mind to the question to be decided could have arrived at it. Although it might be thought that irrationality sat uneasily with competence to decide, panic, indecisiveness and irrationality in themselves did not as such amount to incompetence but might be symptoms or evidence of incompetence. The graver the consequences of the decision the commensurately greater the level of competence was required to take the decision.
- A person lacked capacity if some impairment or disturbance of mental functioning rendered the person unable to make a decision whether to consent to or refuse treatment.
- Temporary factors such as confusion, shock, fatigue, pain or drugs might completely erode capacity but only if such factors were operating to such a degree that the ability to decide was absent.
- Another such influence might be panic induced by fear. Again careful scrutiny of the evidence was necessary because fear of an operation might be a rational reason for refusal to undergo it. Fear might also, however, paralyse the will and thus destroy the capacity to make a decision'.

In addition, she noted that:

- 'Best interests are not limited to medical best interests.'
- 'On the present state of the English law the submission that the court should consider and weigh in the balance the rights of the unborn child were untenable', and rejected prior suggestions that the rights of the unborn child might be taken into consideration as a method of overriding a mother's refusal of treatment.

| Case | *NHS Trust A v M; NHS Trust B v H* [2001] 2 WLR 942 |
|---|---|
| Consideration | Does the withdrawal of non-futile medical treatment render doctors liable for causing an incompetent patients death, thus breaching their human rights? |
| Facts | Hospital Trusts A and B sought declarations that it was legal to discontinue artificial hydration and nutrition to two patients, Mrs M and Mrs H, applications which were supported by the relatives and hospital staff, but opposed by an unincorporated organisation called ALERT. |
| Decision | The declarations were granted. |
| Ratia | Having considered Articles 2, 3 and 8 of the Human Rights Act, 1998 (HRA), precedents set in *Bland*, concerning doctors' duties with regard to the withdrawal of life-saving medical treatment, were not altered. |

| Case | *Paton v British Pregnancy Advisory Service Trustees* [1978] 2 All ER 987; *Paton v UK* [1981] 3 EHRR 408 |
|---|---|
| Consideration | Do fathers, or anyone, have the right to prevent a woman from having an abortion? |
| Facts | Mr Paton sought an injunction to restrain the defendants from carrying out an abortion on his wife (the second defendant) without his consent. |
| Decision | All decisions went against Mr Paton. |
| Ratia | • Fathers, as fathers, have no right to any say in the destiny of any child that they have conceived.<br>• Fathers may not determine what medical interventions that mothers may choose to undergo or refuse.<br>• Fathers, as next friends of the foetus, have no right to any say in the destiny of any child.<br>• These decisions are in accordance with the European Convention on Human Rights (particularly Articles 2 and 8). |

| Case | *Pearce v United Bristol Healthcare NHS Trust* (1998) 48 BMLR 118 (CA) |
|---|---|
| Consideration | What is the standard of information required in relation to the risk of a procedure in order to defend a claim in negligence? |
| Facts | Mrs Pearce was expecting her sixth child. Two weeks after her due date, her obstetrician advised against medical induction of labour, contrary to Mrs Pearce's request. The baby died *in utero*. Mrs Pearce claimed negligence on the part of the obstetrician for failing to advise her of the small additional risk of stillbirth attached to waiting for the onset of natural labour. |
| Decision | • The trial judge dismissed the claim.<br>• Mrs Pearce's appeal was dismissed by the Court of Appeal. |
| Ratia | *Pearce* is a synthesis of *Sidaway* and *Bolitho*, in that the legal standard of duty in all cases, whether concerned with treatment, diagnosis or disclosure of information, depends on the significance of the risk to a reasonable patient: 'if there is a significant risk which would affect the judgement of a reasonable patient, then in the normal course it is the responsibility of the doctor to inform the patient of that significant risk, if the information is needed so that the patient can determine for himself or herself as to what course he or she should adopt'. |

| Case | *Pretty v Director of Public Prosecutions and Secretary of State for the Home Department* [2001] UKHL 61 |
|---|---|
| Consideration | Does a person's 'right to life' similarly afford a 'right to die'? Are the rights of a terminally ill patient breached by refusing the patient's demand to have their life shortened? |
| Facts | Dianne Pretty, 42-year old, sought an undertaking that the Director of Public Prosecutions would not prosecute her husband Brian under Section 2(1) of the Suicide Act 1961, for aiding and abetting a suicide, if he assisted the death of his wife, who was suffering from motor neurone disease and was disabled to the extent that she was unable to take her own life. |
| Decision | Her application was denied in all UK courts, and by the European Court of Human Rights. |
| Ratia | • The decisions of the UK courts affirmed that aiding and abetting a suicide remained a criminal act in the UK, effectively excluding any move towards legalised euthanasia.<br>• The 'right to life' described by Article 2 of the HRA, reflects the sanctity of life, and does not extend to a right to choose when to die.<br>• Doctors were not torturing Mrs Pretty or subjecting her to cruel, inhumane or degrading treatment by keeping her alive (contrary to Article 3 of the HRA), because her suffering resulted from her illness rather than from any medical action.<br>• The right to respect for private and family life (Article 8) relates to the conduct of *life*, rather than death. |

| Case | *Sidaway v Board of Governors of Bethlem Royal Hospital and the Maudsley Hospital* [1985] 1 AC 871 |
|---|---|
| Consideration | What is the standard of information required of a doctor in order to defend a claim of negligence? |
| Facts | Mrs Sidaway suffered considerable disability and paralysis after a cervical microdiscectomy. She alleged that the surgeon had failed to disclose or explain to her the risks inherent in the operation that he had advised (1–2% risk of damage to the spinal column or nerve roots), and that, but for his negligent non-disclosure, she would have not undergone the procedure. |
| Decision | Her claim for negligence was dismissed by the High Court, the Court of Appeal, and by a three to two majority in the House of Lords. |
| Ratia | • *Sidaway* affirmed the *Bolam* principle in relation to the provision of information that is that a doctor would not be negligent if his failure to inform a patient of the risks of surgery was in accordance with practices accepted at the time as proper by a responsible body of medical opinion, even though other doctors may have informed the patient of the risks.<br>• However, *Sidaway* confirmed that the material risks of a procedure must be disclosed.<br>• The case confirmed the 'therapeutic privilege' of doctors to withhold psychologically damaging information from patients, but that the doctor may be called on to justify his decision to withhold information.<br>• The ratio of *Sidaway* may change in future, in light of *Chester v Afshar*. |

| Case | *ReT (adult: refusal of medical treatment)* [1992] 4 All ER 649 |
|---|---|
| Consideration | What is meant by voluntariness in legally valid consent? |
| Facts | Miss T, 34 weeks pregnant, was admitted to hospital 3 days after a road traffic accident, complaining of chest pains. Miss T was not a Jehovah's Witnesses, but shortly after a period of time spent with her fervent Jehovah's Witnesses mother, she refused any blood transfusion. Her condition worsened towards pneumonia and premature onset of labour. She consented to caesarian section, but it was not made clear to her that blood transfusion may be required. The baby was stillborn. Miss T was admitted to intensive therapy unit (ITU) with a lung abscess. A declaration sought by the hospital was granted, allowing blood transfusion in her best interests. |
| Decision | An appeal against the first decision was dismissed by the Court of Appeal. |
| Ratia | • Undue third party influence (in this case the religious beliefs of T's mother) may vitiate valid consent or refusal.<br>• Treatment in the absence of consent should take place out of necessity, and in the patient's best interests.<br>• No one may consent to treatment on behalf of an incompetent adult. |

## QUESTIONS

The following questions have been designed to stimulate discussion amongst readers, or groups of readers, and cover a range of issues that are encountered in contemporary medical practice.

1  What articles of the HRA have relevance to the provision of perioperative care? Address your answer specifically to the provision of postoperative pain relief, consent issues in the under-16s, and the withdrawal of life sustaining treatment.

2 Are doctors ethically obliged to participate in the rationing of healthcare?

3 'Smokers should contribute to the cost of their healthcare'. Discuss.

4 Sally, a 17-year-old anorexic who has run away from home, presents for emergency appendicectomy. Consider the potential problems of consent inherent in this case.

5 'Valid consent is never true consent'. Discuss.

6 Is conscientious objection an acceptable part of medical practice?

7 'There is no such thing as a dignified death'. Discuss, with relevance to euthanasia.

8 How might you change perioperative practices at your hospital in order that they become more compliant with the HRA?

9 Ada, who is 94, demented and living in a nursing home, has fallen out of bed and fractured her right neck of femur, necessitating operative repair. Her son refuses to sign a consent form allowing the surgery to continue, because he says that his mother never would have consented to surgery if she knew in advance that she would be in such a physical and mental condition. Advise the orthopaedic surgeon about issues of consent in this patient.

10 During a bilateral hernia repair on 24-year-old Mr A, Mr Y is called away to treat a gunshot wound in casualty. Dr X, his senior house officer (SHO), continues the procedure, although it is only the fifth hernia repair he has performed. A year later, Mr A, who had been a sperm donor whilst at university, is diagnosed with azoospermia – and his fiancee breaks off their engagement as a result. Mr A suspects the hernia repair may have something to do with it, and consults his solicitor. Advise the hospital's lawyer on how to respond to Mr A's solicitor.

11 Jane has Huntington's chorea. Having seen her father die with the condition as a child, she is understandably nervous about developing the end stages of the disease. She does not want to be treated if dementia eventuates, and writes a living will forbidding CPR if it is ever needed in future. A week later she is struck by lightning, and rushed to hospital by her husband. During CPR, the Accident and Emergency doctor finds a copy of the will in her purse, but decides that Jane does not intend that CPR should not be attempted under the current circumstances, also noting that the will does not appear to have been witnessed. Unfortunately, Jane suffers severe hypoxic brain damage, requiring prolonged ventilation. She develops ventilator-associated pneumonia, and bed sores which break down, requiring surgical debridement. During

the procedure, she has an asystolic arrest. Despite CPR, Jane dies.
Discuss some of the legal issues raised by this case.

12  Latisha, a 15-year old, presents with an antepartum haemorrhage at
    38 weeks. She is extremely needle phobic. Her mother, from whom
    Latisha has so far concealed the pregnancy, is a Jehovah's
    Witnesses, who refuses to allow blood to be given to her daughter.
    Unravel the medicolegal problems that arise in this instance.

13  Giving examples, discuss to what extent does UK law recognise the
    wishes of patients' relatives in making treatment decisions? Do you
    agree with the current law? What changes would you make?

14  Is informed consent 'a fairy story' in the case of perioperative
    medicine?

15  'Pregnancy only confers legal rights on the mother'. Discuss.

16  If fear, pain and drug administration render patients only partially
    autonomous, can valid consent ever be given in the perioperative
    setting?

17  Tracey, a 21-year-old model, undergoes a negative laparoscopy, for
    which she is given a general anaesthetic. Unfortunately, she develops
    phlebitis on the dorsum of her right hand, at a cannula site. The
    wound breaks down, and despite antibiotic therapy, she is left with
    a scar. Tracey sues the hospital and the anaesthetist involved, saying
    that she can no longer pursue a career in modelling – she was due
    to shoot for Vogue soon after the operation. She alleges that she
    did not know that general anaesthesia required her 'to have a
    drip', and did not complain at the time of its insertion because of
    the effects of premedicant sedation. Does she have a case?

18  Are doctors deontologists?

19  Panjit, a 46-year-old mother of six undergoes total abdominal
    hysterectomy. During the procedure, the surgeon (Mr B) notes
    that her appendix is inflamed and removes it. Unfortunately,
    within 24 h postoperatively, Panjit develops peritonitis. Intravenous
    antibiotics are only commenced after 48 h, when her care is
    transferred to Mr C, a general surgeon. She undergoes laparotomy;
    however, the appendicectomy site is intact and no other pathology
    is noted. There is no faecal soiling. She is transferred to ITU,
    where despite the heroic attempts at treatment, she dies 3 days
    later of multiple organ failure. Autopsy reveals a small right
    subphrenic collection of pus, but nothing else in the abdomen.
    Panjit's husband sues the hospital, Mr B and Mr C for negligence.
    How might the courts view his claim?

20  'English Law is overly deferential to the pharmaceutical industry'.
    Discuss.

21 'The General Medical Council (GMC) no longer provides adequate protection for the public against the incompetence of doctors and nurses'. Discuss.

22 Jane, a surgical secretary, overhears Mr Q's telephone discussion with an occupational health physician. Mr Q is concerned about possible human immunodeficiency virus (HIV) transmission, after sustaining a needlestick injury during an operation on a Mr Smith. Jane is a close friend of Mr Smith's wife, and tells her that Mr Q thinks that Mr Smith has HIV. Two months later the hospital is sued by Mr Smith, both for the psychological trauma of his wife divorcing him (citing infidelity), and loss of earnings (his wife telling Mr Smith's boss that he had HIV). Advise the hospital on how to deal with Mr Smith's claim.

23 The legal regulation of research in the UK is woefully inadequate'. Discuss.

24 'For consent to be truly valid, there should be full disclosure of all known risks and consequences of a proposed treatment'. Discuss.

25 'If you can pay for healthcare, you should pay for healthcare'. Discuss

26 'Access to health records is a privilege, and not a right, in the UK'. Discuss.

27 'The law relating to medical negligence is unnecessarily deferential towards doctors in the UK'. Discuss.

28 Examine critically the extent to which the public interest should justify the disclosure of confidential information.

29 Dr Finkelstein is in love with Kate, an ITU nurse. However, Dr Finkelstein knows that he is a carrier for cystic fibrosis (CF). His uncle had the condition, and Dr Finkelstein is petrified that his children will develop CF. In passing conversation, Kate mentions a history of CF in her family – she was tested for the gene 10 years ago, at the hospital at which they both work, but was never informed of the result. Dr Finkelstein looks up the result of Kate's test on the hospital's computerised result service, and, horrified to find that she is also a carrier, he breaks off their relationship without giving any reason. Distraught, Kate seeks comfort in the arms of Dr Finkelstein's twin brother. Dr Finkelstein tells his brother of Kate's carrier status, and Kate is cast into the romantic wilderness for a second time, although Dr Finkelstein's brother at least tells her that he cannot marry her for fear that their children would have CF. Kate sues the hospital, Dr Finkelstein and his brother for breach of confidentiality in relation to her medical records. Advise the defendants on whether they have a case to answer.

30  Ludmilla, 15, alleges that Stanislav raped her 6 months previously. She was too frightened to tell anyone at the time, but now wants an abortion. Stanislav denies rape, and, keen to become a father, objects to Ludmilla's abortion request, saying that, as a father, he has rights in the matter. The obstetric registrar, having been threatened by Stanislav, refuses to perform the abortion, citing conscientious objection. Discuss the legal complexities of this case in relation to current UK abortion legislation.

31  Mr F is asked by Loaded Industries Inc. to trial a new type of silicone-coated, femoral intramedullary nail. After fitting 25 of these, Loaded Industries Inc. reviews his results as part of their post-marketing surveillance. The company is appalled to discover that Mr F has been inserting the nails upside-down, placing them at significant risk of mechanical failure; however, there have been no complaints from the patients, and Loaded Industries Inc. decide not to warn the patients for fear of compensation claims. Five years later, 70% of the patients have developed incapacitating aches and pains. Coincidently, a publication in a leading medical journal suggests that patients with silicone-impregnated prostheses are at a markedly greater risk of developing incapacitating aches and pains. Mr F's patients form an action group, and attempt to sue Mr F, the hospital and Loaded Industries Inc. Loaded Industries Inc.'s previous cover-up is brought to light during preliminary enquiries. Advise all three defendants on the legal liabilities arising in this case.

32  Stiff, Crime and Leech'em have just developed yet another COX-2 inhibitor (lodacoxib) for use as a postoperative analgesic. This one, however, is claimed to have even more 'miraculous properties' than other similar drugs: studies in rats have shown that lodacoxib not only reduces pain after femoral fracture, but also appears to relieve subjective symptoms of dementia. Smith, Crime and Leech'em approach you, proposing a randomised, controlled trial to test these effects against the brand-leading drug, anothacoxib. In order to test the anti-dementing properties of the drug, they would like to enrol aged demented patients who require surgical femoral repair. Discuss some of the legal implications that arise from their proposition.

33  Should the young have improved access to healthcare, in comparison to the elderly?

34  Moonchild, an 18-year old, grew up in a community run by the Loonians, a bizarre cult that shuns modern medicine and counts among its beliefs the idea that implanted surgical devices allow the

subject to be monitored by the government. After a road-accident, the unfortunate Moonchild suffers severe head and leg injuries. Doctors at the attending hospital are unaware that Moonchild is a Loonian. In the absence of next of kin, they quickly operate on Moonchild's legs in an attempt to avoid amputation; intramedullary nails inserted into both tibiae seem to do the trick, and Moonchild is taken to ITU. When her mother, also a Loonian, is informed of what has happened to her daughter, she angrily demands that the intramedullary nails are removed forthwith. The doctors refuse. Unfortunately, Moonchild's condition does not improve. She is eventually declared 'brain dead' after 4 days. Her mother refuses organ donation, and indicates that she will consult solicitors over her daughter's treatment. Prepare a response to the possible contents of such a letter, on behalf of the hospital.

35 Patients are legally dead after the first set of brainstem death tests, rendering any further treatment not in the (incompetent) patient's best interests. Are doctors, therefore, legally justified in continuing intensive therapy: (a) until a second set of tests is performed, and (b) until the patient undergoes organ harvest?

36 To what extent does English law recognise a 15-year old's right to die?

37 If the UK adopts an 'opt out' scheme for organ donation, should those who opt out of the scheme be denied organ transplants?

38 'The court's opinion should always be sought before medical treatment is withdrawn'. Discuss this opinion with reference to UK common law.

39 'Living wills provide adequate protection of an unconscious patient's autonomy'. Discuss, giving examples, in relation to current UK law.

40 'Whistleblowing should be considered a virtue in the modern NHS'. Is it?

# Index